D1487057

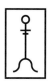

# WITHDRAWN
No longer the property of the
Boston Public Library.
Sale of this material benefits the Library

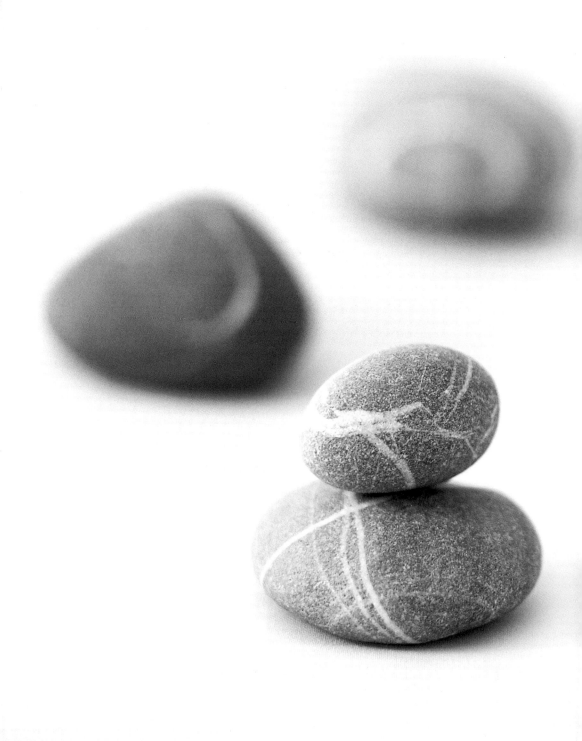

# The weekend
# HEALER

**More than a Dozen 3-Day Plans to Relax,
Relieve Stress, and Re-energize**

## jane alexander

A Fireside Book
Published by Simon & Schuster
New York London Toronto Sydney Singapore

# a gaia original

Books from Gaia celebrate the vision of Gaia, the self-sustaining living Earth, and seek to help its readers live in greater personal and planetary harmony.

| | |
|---|---|
| Editorial | Pip Morgan |
| Design | Sara Mathews |
| Photography | Craig Robertson, Gus Filgate, and Paul Forrester |
| Production | Lyn Kirby |
| Direction | Joss Pearson |
| | Patrick Nugent |

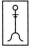

FIRESIDE
Rockefeller Center
1230 Avenue of the Americas
New York, NY 10020

Copyright © 2002 by Gaia Books Limited
Text Copyright © 2002 by Jane Alexander
All rights reserved, including the right of reproduction in whole or in part in any form.

FIRESIDE and colophon are registered trademarks of Simon & Schuster, Inc.

Manufactured in Singapore

10 9 8 7 6 5 4 3 2 1

Library of Congress Cataloging-in-Publication Data
Alexander, Jane.
    The weekend healer : more than a dozen 3-day plans to relax, relieve stress, and re-energize/Jane Alexander.
      p.  cm.
    "A Fireside book."
    Includes bibliographical references.
    ISBN 0-7432-2438-8
    1. Health. 2. Stress management. 1. Title

RA776 .A3735 2002
613--dc21                          2001040890

For information regarding special discounts for bulk purchases, please contact Simon & Schuster Special Sales at 1-800-456-6798 or business@simonandschuster.com

*For Jane Rayson –*
*a great weekender and*
*a great friend*

## Author acknowledgments

Huge thanks to Pip Morgan and Sara Mathews who have worked so hard on this project. A vast number of experts have helped me over the years but, in brief, I would like to thank the following: Virginie Host, Fiona Arrigo, the staff at Tyringham naturopathic clinic, Sue Weston, Angela Hope-Murray, Ian and Carole Heywood, Susan Lever, Sarah Dening, Richard Lanham, Jane Mayers, Sarah Shurety, Karen Kingston, Denise Linn, Ron Wilgosh, Sheila McCleod, Leo Rutherford, Nicki Skully, Shan, and Kate Roddick.

Love and thanks to my family and friends who share my weekends and make them so special. And a big hug to Judy Chilcote, my agent, with whom I'd like to spend MORE weekends!

## Gaia acknowledgments

Gaia Books would like to thank Lynn Bresler, Elizabeth Wiggans, the models (Rosie Hill, Emily Heap, Raksha Patel, Daniel Del Rio), Sunil Vijayakar for home economy, Thomas Hawes for design assistance, and Will Heap for photographic assistance.

# How to use this book

Come Friday afternoon and we're all looking forward to the same thing: a stress-free, refreshing, and fulfilling weekend. And, of course, we all know how to achieve this – or do we?

*The Weekend Healer* is designed to make sure you do. It provides a broad range of seventeen programs that you can indulge in at home. The whole idea is to help you enjoy your weekend to the full, while at the same time experiencing the positive effects of natural therapies and techniques.

You may have a specific weekend in mind, which is fine. If not, take some time just browsing through the book – is there a weekend that takes your fancy or one which you instinctively feel you need? Another approach is to just sit with your eyes closed and slowly flip through the book until you feel the urge to stop. See which weekend you have landed on and go for it! Or else randomly pick a page number out of the top of your head and see which weekend it lies within.

Once you have chosen your weekend, you need to make preparations. The list at the beginning of each weekend gives a rough idea of the main things you will need. But spend some time reading through the weekend beforehand and figuring out precisely what you will need to make that weekend special. Look at the resources and further reading – the leads you find there may help you to be better prepared. And if you are going to incorporate a treament, a bodywork session, or some time at the gym – don't forget to make a appointment!

Try as far as possible to get in everything you need before the weekend starts. Not just any special "props" but also basics such as food and drink.

I do hope you find these weekends inspiring and exciting. I hope they bring you fresh insights and new ways of looking at yourself, the people you know, and the world around you. Above all, I hope you enjoy them and find them good fun.

*Happy weekending!*

# Contents

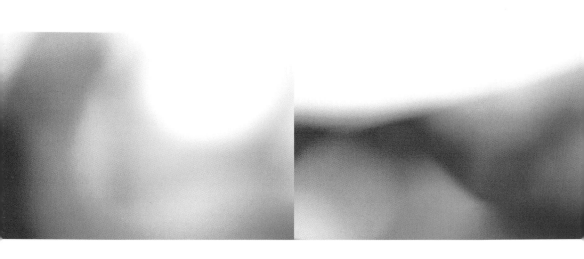

# Introduction

Weekends are special. They are oases of calm in a hectic world, offering "time out" from work and everyday routine. They are times when we can do what we please and be who we want to be. Or so they should be. Too often we waste our weekends in a flurry of chores, in endless shopping trips, or by flopping and "vegging" out in front of the television or watching videos. Don't fall into the wasted weekend trap.

A weekend is just the perfect amount of time for a healing break: an evening followed by two whole days should be time enough to make serious changes in your life or to set up a whole new pattern or even to shift into an entirely new way of living.

## CHOOSING A WEEKEND

This book has seventeen different kinds of weekend so I hope there is one to suit everybody's needs. Each weekend is organized and planned along the lines of a Friday evening, Saturday, and Sunday – this is designed to give you a time frame to work with and an unfolding structure to follow.

If you feel the need to give your body some attention you can spend a weekend making friends with your body (in the Body awareness weekend) or gently detoxing your entire system. If you're lacking in energy then try the Energizing weekend. If you need some pampering then go for the Beauty weekend. If you need to rebalance your wellbeing then try the Ayurvedic weekend.

If it's your mind and emotions that need a workout, you could opt for one of the weekends in Part Two – learning how to get in touch with your subconscious; or rethinking your life; or getting out of a rut. Everyone in a couple should try the Relationships weekend at least once, if not regularly!

The wellbeing of our spirits, souls, and inner lives is all too often ignored in our busy lives and so, in Part Three, you will find several weekends that can help you to redress the balance – teaching key concepts and practices, such as meditation, prayer, ritual, and altar-making. And if you have ever wondered about practices such as shamanism, the Tarot, or the Qabalah, then you can get a taster by following the weekends that introduce their essential elements.

The last part of the book provides you with ideas for welcoming and celebrating Spring, Summer, Autumn, and Winter. Our ancestors would have enjoyed a cycle of festivals and rituals to mark the changing year. Here, you will find weekends to tie in with the four major seasons. They will help your mind, body, and spirit attune to the shifting energy patterns of the year and so address the major issues and changes each season might bring.

At the end of the book there are two key yoga practices – the Sun Salutation for the beginning of the day and the Moon Salutation for the evening. These feature in several of the weekends and will make a welcome addition to your everyday life.

## MAKING THE WEEKENDS WORK

Before embarking on a weekend there are some important things to sort out first so that the weekend works better and runs more smoothly. Make sure you inform your family and friends what you are doing – and explain that you won't be able to rush off and do things in the usual way.

If you're sharing your house then ask if other people would be willing to help out by giving you peace and quiet when you need it; by clearing up their mess so you don't have to do it; taking messages for you on the phone; leaving you the bathroom free for your evening bathing ritual – or whatever.

If you live alone – or have planned your weekend so you will be alone (a great option) – then you might consider putting a special message on your answerphone and a note on the door explaining you're busy.

## PEACE AND QUIET

Not all the weekends in this book call for absolute solitude – in fact, many of them are very sociable! But there are a few, in particular the spiritual ones, that do require peace and quiet.

For example, you really should not be interrupted in the middle of shamanic journeying or Qabalistic pathworking. So when you are engaged in such rituals, do make it clear to anyone around that you MUST NOT be disturbed for the duration of the ritual. Coming very swiftly out of a deep journeying ritual can be very disturbing to the psyche and could result in a rotten headache or a feeling of general dis-ease.

If you ARE jolted out of one of these rituals, you must ask for five minutes to "recollect" yourself and sit quietly, breathing deeply. Apologize to any inner world beings you may have been communicating with and swiftly but surely bring yourself through the returning steps of the ritual. Remember to stamp your feet and become fully grounded.

## BE FLEXIBLE

The suggestions for each weekend are just that – suggestions. Don't feel you have to rigidly follow them as if they were a doctor's prescription! Be flexible and intuitive.

If you really dislike art, for example, and the weekend suggests you get out your paints and crayons to visualize your feelings, you have two options: either you decide that you might discover something interesting by working through your distaste and just go for it; or you pick something similar from another weekend (maybe some movement, music, or dialoguing with yourself).

On a more practical level, you may find that the instructions in one of the weekends recommends you take a bath of some kind – but how can you as you only have a shower! Always try to adapt the instructions to your personal circumstances – for instance, you can put drops of an aromatherapy oil on to some unbleached muslin cloth and tie it around the shower head.

The instructions for some exercises, such as the Sun Salutation, can consist of a number of steps and seem complicated. You may therefore find them quite hard to read and follow at the same time. A good suggestion for making it easier would be to record the instructions on an audio cassette and then play them back as you do the exercises. Remember to put in lots of pauses to give you time to take up positions.

## SAFETY FIRST

Everything in this book is inherently safe. I have tried all the exercises myself and I use many of them on a regular basis. However, they ARE powerful and many of them work at a very deep level, both on the body and the psyche.

If you suffer from any physical health problems, or other medical conditions or concerns, I would firmly advise you to check with your physician before performing any of the exercises in this book. It makes good sense because then you will be able to relax more fully knowing that you won't be doing yourself any harm.

## DEALING WITH THE UNEXPECTED

Every weekend – even the very physical body ones – will also work deeply on a psychological level. Don't be surprised or afraid if some exercises bring up old or unexpected emotions or memories. You may find some of the emotions unsettling or downright uncomfortable.

For the most part, I believe we only bring to conscious awareness those issues with which we are ready to deal. If you find yourself feeling uncomfortable, stop doing the exercise and spend some time breathing deeply to calm yourself before returning to the work.

If you feel the emotion is simply too much, stop the exercise altogether and make yourself a cup of tea and do something very ordinary and mundane, such as watching the television or listening to the radio.

When you feel calm, you might want to talk your experience over with a friend. You might also consider finding a qualified therapist to work with. I firmly believe that if an unpleasant emotion or memory emerges, it is asking for your attention. But if the emotion is very painful, do turn to a professional for help and advice.

## IMPORTANT

*The techniques in this book should be used at the reader's sole discretion. Always observe the cautions given in the text and consult your doctor if you are in any doubt about a medical condition.*

# **Part one:** bodycare

*How much time do you devote to your body during the week? Even with the best intentions, it can be tough to look after your physical self while you're juggling work, family, and the daily demands of the world. Often you end up eating the wrong kind of food or hurriedly consuming fast food or pre-prepared meals on the run or on your lap. You sit slumped over a computer all day or torture your body on long car journeys. You barely have time to think about activity and exercise.*

*A weekend is the perfect time for a body workout. It's a great opportunity to break out of bad routines, to try new diets and exercise programmes, to pamper and preen yourself. The weekends in this part are all designed to make you feel much better in your body. If you're feeling totally out of touch with your body, reacquaint yourself with the Body Awareness weekend: it's a great place to start, a natural forerunner to all the other weekends. If you aren't aware of your body, you can't possibly move further into the realm of mind and spirit.*

*Other weekends in this part will help you to probe deeper into your mind-body connection and provide a wake-up call for the Self. You can choose to boost your energy levels, detox your entire system, or pamper yourself with a total beauty weekend. You also get a taster of the incredible Indian practice of Ayurveda – a complete system for total health and wellbeing.*

*You may find the effects of these weekends will extend further and be made part of your everyday life. Simple lifestyle changes can be enormously effective and even the tiniest shifts can make you look and feel much better.*

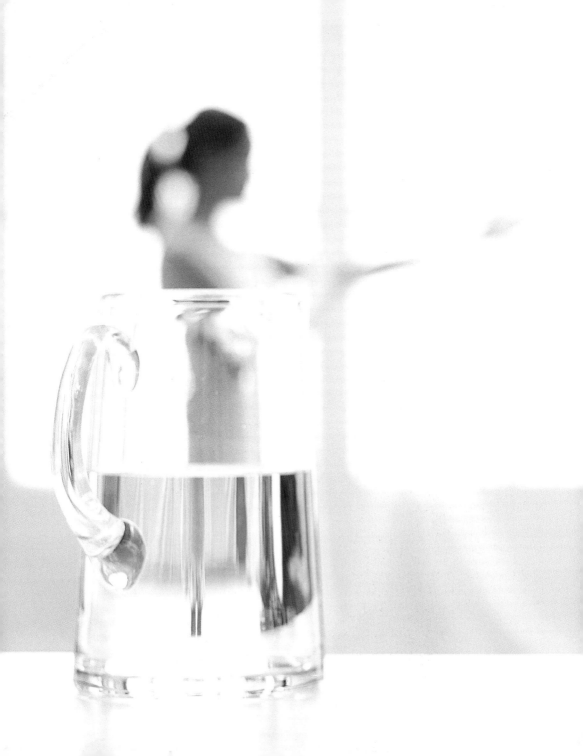

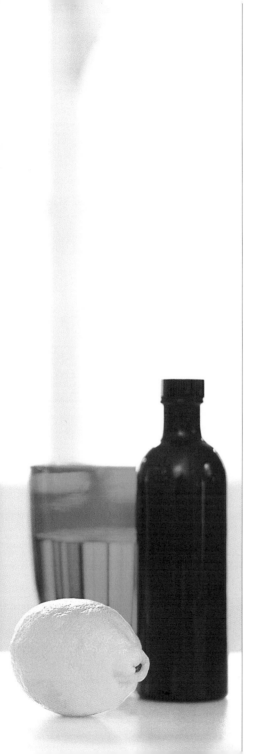

# Body awareness

*What kind of relationship do you have with your body? Are you good friends with each other? Are you indifferent acquaintances or, even worse, sworn enemies? Few of us are really in touch deep down with our bodies and the consequences can range from niggling aches and pains to a chronic disease. This weekend will help you redefine your relationship with your body in a way that will set you on the road to better health.*

WHAT YOU'LL NEED:
- *Healthy eating foods (see page 17)*
- *10 pints (6 litres) mineral water*
- *Essential oils: lemon, geranium, lavender, and Roman chamomile*
- *Sweet almond oil*
- *Walnut Bach flower remedy*
- *Paper and crayons or paints*

# Friday evening TALK TO YOUR BODY

We rarely ask our bodies what they need or want. So this evening and on Saturday and Sunday morning sit down quietly and start a dialogue with your body. Ask:

✦ What it needs right now – water; food (if so, what food?); a good stretch; exercise; rest; sleep?

✦ What it would like to do now?

✦ What changes it would like you to make in general: change of diet; more, less, or different exercise; stress relief; more rest?

Follow your body's wishes as wholeheartedly as you can. Make a plan of how to adapt your lifestyle to help your body with what it needs. If this is difficult, imagine what your body MIGHT say, were it to know. Play with the idea – you may be surprised at what emerges.

### SHOWER RITUAL

Start the evening with a refreshing shower ritual:

**1.** Put a couple of drops of lemon oil (which is refreshing and promotes self-awareness) on a wash cloth or loofah.

**2.** As you wash each part of your body, focus and bring awareness to that part. Affirm to yourself that, this weekend, you will treat your body with kindness.

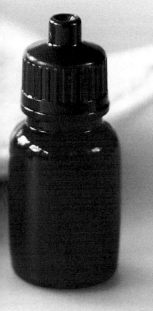

## HOW DOES EATING MAKE YOU FEEL?

Tonight, eat your usual kind of supper but become aware of what you are eating and drinking.

✦ How does it taste? How does it feel in your mouth?

✦ How do you feel as you eat?

✦ How do you feel after your meal? Ten minutes later?

✦ Become aware of how your body enjoys (or doesn't!) the food you feed it. Does your body like its diet? Does the food give you the right combination of energy and peace? Do you sleep well after eating?

### HEALTHY EATING

*Try to eat food that is organic, grown locally and in its natural season, and provides your body with the best possible nutrition.*

✦ *Fresh fruit, vegetables: five portions daily.*

✦ *Complex carbohydrates: whole or unrefined grains (brown rice, oats), wholemeal pasta and bread, potatoes.*

✦ *Protein: legumes, nuts, lean white meat, fish (particularly oily fish), soy bean products.*

✦ *Flavour your food with herbs and spices.*

✦ *3 pints (2 litres) fresh mineral water daily.*

✦ *Cut down on: alcohol, caffeine, salt, sugar, artificial sweeteners; "junk" and fast food, pre-prepared meals; smoked meats, sausages, red meat, full-fat dairy produce, and fried foods.*

# Saturday GETTING IN TOUCH

Spend at least 20 minutes on this exercise when you wake up. It will help you become more conscious of how your body feels. Spend the morning doing gentle exercise.

**1.** Wear no clothes, or only loose-fitting nightwear, and lie on your back on the floor.

**2.** Become aware of your body. Feel the floor underneath – notice where your body touches it and where it doesn't.

**3.** Focus your attention on your feet. How do your toes feel? Your heels? Are your feet hot or cold? Light or heavy? Is there any difference between the two feet?

**4.** Work up your legs, asking the same questions of your ankles, your calves, your knees, thighs, and hips. Move to your buttocks, belly, abdomen, chest, and shoulders.

**5.** Concentrate on your back. How does your spine feel? Do you notice any difference between the lower, middle, and upper regions of your spine? How is your neck? Continue down your arms, wrists, and hands.

**6.** Finally move to your face and head. Are you holding tension in your jaw? Is there a difference between one side of the face and the other? One eye and the other? Your ears? How does your scalp feel? Your hair?

**DAWN AFFIRMATION**
*Take three drops of the Walnut Bach flower remedy in a glass of mineral water. Walnut helps you to make changes and to break with your old, unhealthy, unhelpful habits. Affirm to yourself as you lie in bed that your aim this weekend is to learn to listen to your body's needs and to be kinder and gentler with it.*

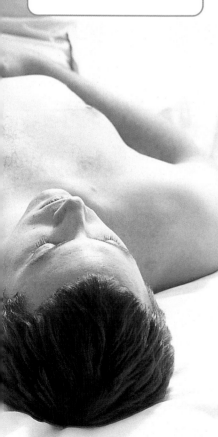

**A TOUCHING AFTERNOON**
*Do you suffer from touch deprivation? Is your body simply not stroked, rubbed, massaged, and touched enough? Organize a session of bodywork – try Thai massage, aromatherapy, shiatsu, or Chinese tui na massage. You may release old hurts and memories.*

## THE ART OF GOOD BREATHING

Breathing well puts you in touch with your body and is an invaluable tool for good health.

**1.** Lie comfortably on the floor and bring your feet close in to your buttocks. Place the soles of the feet together, hands resting gently on your abdomen. (If this feels uncomfortable then put cushions under your knees.) The posture stretches the lower abdomen and so enhances the breathing process.

**2.** Breathe in with a slow, smooth inhalation through your nostrils, feeling your abdomen expand and contract.

**3.** Exhale slowly and steadily through your nose, noticing your fingers touching as your abdomen flattens.

**4.** Pause for a second or two. Repeat this inhalation and exhalation, becoming conscious of the movement of the breath down through your chest and abdomen. Continue at your own pace for around five minutes.

**5.** If you feel comfortable with this you can extend the breath so it comes up from the abdomen into the chest as you inhale. This provides a longer, deeper breath.

**6.** Finally, bring your knees together and gently stretch out the legs. Relax on the ground for a few minutes.

## BATH AND MASSAGE

Finish your day with a long, luxurious bath (add two drops each of lavender and Roman chamomile oils to relax and foster acceptance). Afterwards, massage yourself with a blend of four drops each of the above oils in four teaspoons (15–20 ml) of sweet almond oil. Pay attention to each part of your body, spending more time on the parts which are sore or stressed. You don't need perfect technique – just a willingness to touch and connect with your body.

# Sunday GOING DEEPER

As you become more aware of your body affirm to yourself that it's satisfying. Don't dismiss doubts or problems but quietly think the issues through. You may find it useful to write down your thoughts and irritations.

## LET YOUR BODY CHOOSE

Repeat the Saturday's body awareness routine and then check what your body wants to do today. It might ask to:

✦ Walk: don't march, be aware of how you are walking, and what you are seeing, hearing, feeling around you.

✦ Sit under a tree: to muse, meditate, read, or dream.

✦ Exercise: maybe a bike ride, a swim, a session at the gym, or an aerobics class.

✦ Enjoy another massage: try a different one. Or you could find a friend and trade massages.

✦ Play sport: which sports did you enjoy at school? Join a team or a club; or just play a sport with your children.

✦ Try mind-body exercises, such as yoga, Pilates, chi kung, or tai chi.

✦ Try new ways of cooking and eating. Low-fat and vegetarian cooking are good choices; so is eating macrobiotically. Enhance your cooking habits by joining a healthy cooking class, or simply look for a different kind of cookbook – one you've never tried before.

✦ See a natural healthcare practitioner: your body might be crying out for a dose of homeopathy, acupuncture, herbalism, nutritional therapy, Ayurveda, or reflexology.

## FOLLOW YOUR BODY'S ORDERS

This afternoon, learn more about your body with movement and art. Make sure you will not be disturbed and don't be afraid to follow your urges – this isn't about "proper" dancing or "good" art.

**1.** Take off your shoes and socks and walk around the room, becoming aware of how your body relates to it. Notice how your feet feel on the floor. Notice how your arms might want to stretch out.

**2.** Stop for a moment and balance firmly on both feet. Feel your body relax into your pelvis. Feel your pelvis as a bowl which supports your body. Bring your awareness here and feel how it wants to move.

**3.** Really listen to what your body wants. It might feel like throwing itself around the room; it might want to sway gently; it might want to curl up in a ball.

**4.** If you do stop moving, it might just be a pause. Be ready for a movement and await your body's orders.

**5.** When your body has expressed itself fully, use crayons (or paints) to let your hands inscribe how your body feels or what message it is giving. Your drawing doesn't have to be representative – it might just be marks or colours.

**6.** Sit back and look at what you have created. Write down any thoughts that come to mind.

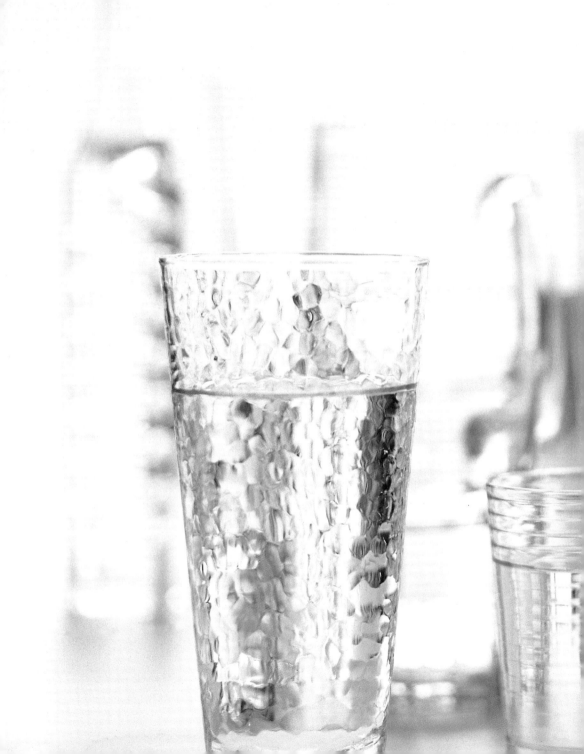

# Detox yourself

*Sometimes you just know you've overdone it! Your mind is sluggish, your body feels uncomfortable, and your energy levels are close to zero. It's time for a detox. This weekend cleanse is gentle and safe (yet still effective) and offers your body a rejuvenating break.*

CAUTION: *Don't detox when pregnant, breastfeeding, menstruating, or with a cold or infection. If you have any medical problems, check with your doctor first.*

### WHAT YOU'LL NEED:
- *Seasonal salads, fruits, and vegetables*
- *Herbal tea: thyme, ginger, peppermint*
- *10 pints (6 litres) of mineral water*
- *Six lemons*
- *Essential oils: rosemary, plus chamomile, pine, or juniper*
- *Epsom salts (or mineral bath)*
- *Natural bristle brush with long handle*
- *Plenty of towels*
- *Candles, inspirational books, music*

# Friday evening GETTING READY

Eat a light diet throughout today in preparation for your weekend. Cut out tea, coffee, and heavy proteins and fat. Drink at least 3 pints (2 litres) of unchilled water. Eat a light supper of salad (with a little olive oil, garlic, lemon, and cider vinegar dressing). From now on, only drink fresh water (warm or room temperature), herbal tea, or ginger tea.

## SKIN BRUSHING
Before you go to bed brush your skin – make sure it's dry so brush before a bath. Skin brushing stimulates the lymphatic system and encourages the expulsion of toxins.
✦ Brush your feet, toes, and soles and then the front and back of your legs (use long, smooth strokes). Always brush upwards and towards the groin.
✦ Brush your buttocks and lower back (as well as you can) using upward strokes.
✦ Brush your hands and arms towards your armpits.
✦ Brush across your shoulders and down the chest towards the heart (avoid your nipples).
✦ Brush the back of your neck with downward strokes.
✦ Using a circular, clockwise motion, brush your abdominal and stomach area.

   Now have a bath to which you have added two drops of rosemary oil. Gradually add cool water until, over a period of about half an hour, the water is quite cold. This further stimulates the lymph.

### DETOX SIDE EFFECTS

*These side effects show you are getting rid of toxins. If you have any concerns, see your doctor.*

+ *A headache*
+ *More, or smellier, sweat*
+ *Fatigue*
+ *Feeling unusual emotions*
+ *A dry mouth*
+ *Spots, pimples, or rashes*
+ *Constipation*

# Saturday SERIOUS CLEANSING

Today, follow a strict mono-diet by eating, or drinking the juice of, one type of fruit or vegetable: either grapes, apples, or carrots. Taking small amounts throughout the day, make sure you chew thoroughly and sip your juice slowly – be conscious of every mouthful.

Start the day with a mug of hot water and freshly squeezed lemon juice. Get out in the fresh air and take a good walk, noticing the world around you.

### THE DETOX BREATH
This powerful breathing exercise will help you eliminate the toxins you are releasing and strengthen and tone your entire system. CAUTION: Do not use if you have a heart condition, high blood pressure, epilepsy, hernia, or if you have any ear, nose, or eye problem.
**1.** Inhale slowly and deeply. Don't overstrain in any way.
**2.** Exhale briskly, as if you were sneezing. As you do, become aware of your abdomen which will naturally tighten and flatten as you exhale.
**3.** Inhale naturally and exhale briskly again.
**4.** Continue this cycle for as long as you feel comfortable. It is very energetic so you may not be able to manage more than a minute to begin with. Do it regularly throughout your weekend and notice how you improve.
**5.** When you finish, return to normal breathing. Notice how you feel.

Follow this exercise, if you can, with a Turkish bath for a steam and massage or else go swimming. You could try a bodywork or massage session: MLD (manual lymphatic drainage) is particularly useful while detoxing as it supports the lymphatic system. But any massage will do you good (ask your therapist to use detoxing oils if you're having aromatherapy).

### EPSOM SALTS BATH

Before turning in for an early night you're going to have a thorough skin-brushing session and then an Epsom salts bath. This induces lots of perspiration so you can sweat out lots of the toxins you are starting to release. CAUTION: Avoid this bath if you have heart trouble, are diabetic, or feel tired and weak. Instead, you can substitute a mineral bath such as a Moor mud bath.

**1.** Dissolve about 16 oz (450 g) of Epsom salts into a warm bath – it shouldn't be too hot.

**2.** Get in and relax for about 20 minutes. Visualize all the toxins coming out from your pores and dissolving in the water. Drink a hot herbal tea (thyme or peppermint) to increase the sweating and replace any fluids you lose.

**3.** Get out carefully as you may feel light headed. Don't rub your body; just swathe yourself in large, warm towels and go to bed, making sure your feet are wrapped up warmly. You'll probably go straight to sleep.

### DETOX YOUR LIFE

This evening, write down how you could detox your life – rather than just your body. What is toxic in your life? Any people? Your work? Your home or the place where you live? What changes would ease your toxic load?

# Sunday COMING CLEAN

During the night you've sweated so sponge yourself down with warm water or shower. Vigorously rub your body dry. Your skin may well be tingling. Drink a cup of hot water with squeezed lemon. Eat fresh fruit salad (see page 153) or, if the weather's cold, stew some fruit (apples, pears plus sultanas, raisins) in a little water instead.

Get some exercise and for lunch eat another fruit salad (mixed seasonal fruit) topped with plain live yogurt. Eat slowly, with awareness, tasting every mouthful.

**DRINK WATER**
*Make sure you drink your 3 pints (2 litres) of water through the day. Try to drink it hot as warm water is supposed to shift toxic matter better than cool water.*

## DETOX MEDITATION

Repeat the detox breathing this afternoon and then spend some time in meditation.

**1.** Sit either on a straight-backed chair or on the floor.
**2.** Check your body to ensure you aren't holding on to tension, especially jaws, shoulders, legs, and buttocks.
**3.** Now focus on your breath. Don't try to change it – just be aware of it. Notice how you breathe in, and how you hold the breath for a moment before exhaling. Then another pause before you inhale. It's a four-step process.
**4.** Follow your breath like this and if your mind starts to wander, don't be angry – just gently bring it back.
**5.** Imagine you're exhaling toxic thoughts and emotions from your body and mind and inhaling new, exciting energy and possibilities.
**6.** When you feel ready, return your focus to the breath.
**7.** Now become aware of your body – of your buttocks sitting on the floor or chair; of your head balancing on your neck; of your shoulders relaxed and heavy.
**8.** Now become aware of the world around you: the sounds, the temperature. Slowly and gently open your eyes and return to normal consciousness.
**9.** Sit for a few minutes. Drink water before getting up.

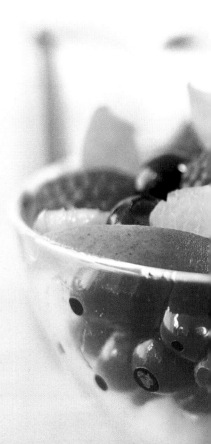

## GO EASY ON YOURSELF

Eat your evening meal early, around 6pm. A simple bowl of steamed vegetables with herbs, spices, and garlic to taste (but no salt). Make a dressing of a teaspoon of olive oil and lemon juice (plus ginger and garlic if you like) and pour over the steamed vegetables. Allow it all to mix together for a few minutes. If you're ravenously hungry, add a portion of boiled brown rice or a baked potato.

Take it easy and pamper yourself this evening. Light some candles and burn an aromatherapy oil (juniper, chamomile, or pine). Curl up with a good book or listen to music.

Check in with your body and see how you feel. Are there parts of the detox you might continue? Give up coffee for good? Drink the hot water and lemon every morning? Devote 20 minutes a day to meditation? Even small changes will help your body feel better.

### CIDER VINEGAR BATH

*Again, plan to get to bed early. Skin brush thoroughly (you should be expert by now). Add two cups of apple cider vinegar to a warm (make sure it's not too hot) bath. Get in and relax for about 15 minutes. This bath is deeply detoxifying. Pat yourself dry and go to bed.*

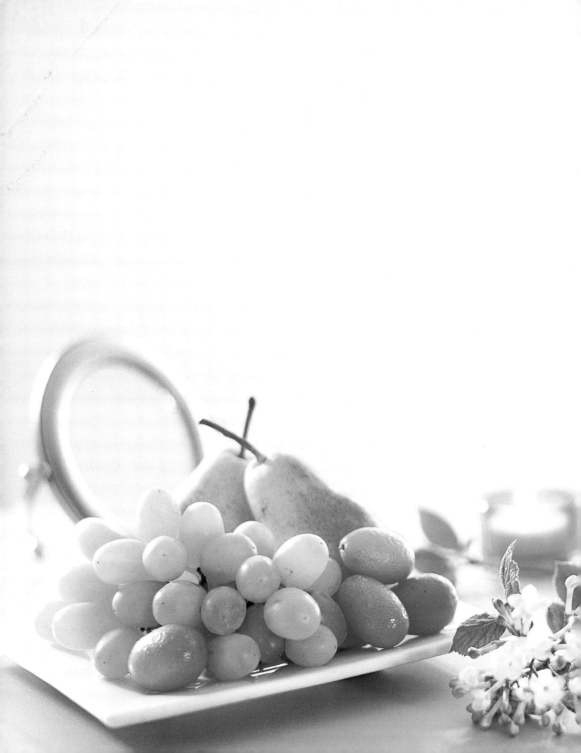

# Beauty weekend

*Who honestly doesn't want to be more beautiful? We may spend a lot of money on fancy cosmetics but few of us really spend time and thought on our bodies. Allowing yourself the luxury of a pampering beauty weekend can make you look – and feel – like a million dollars.*

*WHAT YOU'LL NEED:*
- *Food for beauty (see page 33), including plenty of fruit for eating raw and juicing*
- *Four pints (2.5 litres) fresh, whole milk*
- *Ripe, red cherries; ripe, organic grapes*
- *Large bag of sea salt*
- *25 ml beeswax and 40 ml rosewater*
- *Almond, grapeseed, wheatgerm, coconut oils*
- *Cider vinegar*
- *Wild honey*
- *2 eggs*
- *Green tea*
- *Essential oils: see text for options*
- *Glass jars, sterilized*

# Friday evening MAKE A FRESH START

Look in your make-up bag, your bathroom cabinet, your
cosmetic "shelf" and what do you see? Ten to one, they
are all stuffed full. Yet make-up and cosmetics don't have
an indefinite use-by date: in fact, they can go off quite
quickly. Have a complete turn-out: throw away anything
that is over a year old; anything you don't wear; or
anything that no longer suits you.

If you want to combine this weekend with a detox then
follow the eating guidelines from the Detox weekend (see
pages 22–29). If not, eat a good, healthy diet with an
emphasis on fresh fruit and juice.

Throughout the weekend, try to give your face a break
from make-up – allow it to breathe. Turn your Friday
evening cleansing session into a mini-ritual.

**1.** Light some candles and put on soothing music in the
bathroom. Make sure you have plenty of fluffy towels
ready and warming on the radiator.

**2.** Gently remove all your make-up, ideally with a little
coconut oil – take care not to pull the skin.

**3.** Allow the bath to fill with warm water and then add
4 pints (2.5 litres) of fresh milk and a couple of drops of
chamomile essential oil.

**4.** Mash up ripe organic grapes into a paste (grapes are
toning and nourishing) and apply as a face mask.

**5.** Now gently lower yourself into your milk bath (which
will smooth and moisturize your skin).

**6.** Relax for around 10 minutes then rinse off the mask
and pat your face with the milky water.

**7.** Stay in the bath for another 10 minutes and then get
out and pat your skin dry.

## FOOD FOR BEAUTY

*Good food and drink is an essential part of the beauty equation.*

✦ *Drink 3 pints (2 litres) of fresh mineral water a day.*

✦ *Invest in a juicer and enjoy a variety of juices: orange, grape, papaya, mango, guava, carrot, celery. Drink your juice immediately: sip it slowly, holding it in your mouth for a few seconds before swallowing.*

✦ *Avoid wheat and dairy produce as they tend to clog up the intestines and interfere with nutrient absorption, causing congestion from excess mucus.*

✦ *Complex carbohydrates (potatoes, brown rice, oats, root vegetables, and legumes) should form half your diet.*

✦ *Eat five portions of vegetables and around 2 oz (55 g) of protein (fish, seeds, nuts, and pulses) daily.*

✦ *Use fats in moderation – make sure the oils you buy are cold-pressed and unrefined.*

# Saturday STIMULATE YOUR CIRCULATION

Get moving! If you want a beautiful body, you need to move it! This morning do some exercise and then give yourself a shiatsu facial massage in the afternoon. In the evening take a salt massage bath followed by a wonderful sleep – they don't call it beauty sleep for nothing.

If you're new to exercise visit your local sports or health club and see if anything appeals, or check out gentle yet powerful exercise systems such as yoga or Pilates – they stretch and tone the body without all the huffing and puffing. At the very least go for a good walk or swim. Remember: start and finish any exercise with a series of stretches (your instructor or teacher will show you how).

## SHIATSU FACIAL MASSAGE

Massaging various tsubos (acupressure points) can help to revitalize the face and relieve tension which gives rise to lines. Use either your thumbs or the pads of one or more fingers (experiment with what works best for you). Press for around five seconds on each point – use whatever pressure feels right (some points may be tender but don't press to the point of agony!).

**1.** Close your eyes and gently and softly circle your face with your fingertips.

**2.** Cover your eyes with your palms and relax like this for a few minutes. You can rest your elbows on a table.

**3.** Find the point at the lower edge of each cheekbone, where the bone sticks out. It is usually directly under the middle of each eye. Press on both sides simultaneously.

**4.** Move your fingers to the top of your nose, in the corners of your eyes. Press here with your index fingers.

**5.** Move your fingers out to either side of your eyes (the outer corners nearest your ears). Press at these points.

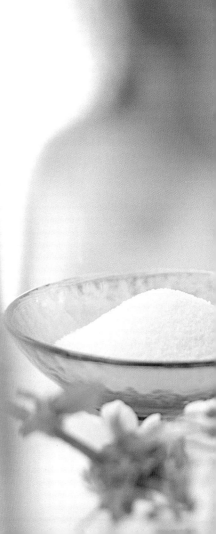

**6.** Find the spot just under your ear lobes, between the bones. Press here (both sides at the same time, as always).
**7.** Move back to the area under your eyes and find the tsubo on the bony edge of the eye sockets. Hold gently.
**8.** Finish by working on your "third eye" spot in between your eyebrows. Press firmly, then apply a little coconut oil and gently, very gently, massage this point in a circular (clockwise) motion. The longer this point is massaged the better – it helps eliminate wrinkles, stimulate circulation, and bring a profound sense of peace.

## SALT MASSAGE BATH

This bath increases circulation and deeply cleanses the skin by sloughing off old cells. CAUTION: Do not use if you have broken skin, high or low blood pressure, or any heart condition.
**1.** Fill the bath with warm water (it shouldn't be too hot) and add a cup or two of sea salt.
**2.** Pour a handful of sea salt into your hand and add some warm water until you have a thick paste.
**3.** Using small, circular movements, massage the paste over your body: start with your neck and shoulders and move slowly down until you reach your feet (don't use on your face and don't rub over nipples).
**4.** Get into the bath and soak for at least 10 minutes.
**5.** Rub yourself dry and have an early night.

# Sunday LOVING ATTENTION

This morning you can make your own cosmetics (see opposite). It's good fun and the beauty of homemade products is that you know exactly what's going into them. But they won't keep as long as store-bought products so keep them in the fridge and use quickly. In the afternoon give your hands and feet some loving attention, followed later by your face, hair, and body.

### FEET AND HANDS MASSAGE
Soak your feet for 15 to 20 minutes in a large bowl of warm water containing 15 ml sea salt, 3 drops almond oil, and 2 to 6 drops peppermint or patchouli oil.

While your feet are soaking, give your hands a treat. Soak them in warm water for about five minutes then massage with a mixture of 10 ml of wheatgerm oil, 5 ml of wild honey, and five drops of lavender oil. Use small, circling movements. Very gently, push back your cuticles and massage your nails with the mixture.

### SOOTHING TREAT
Tonight give your face, hair, and body a soothing treat.
**1.** Prepare a luxurious hair treatment by mixing together two egg yolks, one tablespoon of almond oil, and a drop of tangerine essential oil.
**2.** Moisten your hair and massage the mixture into your scalp and hair. Wrap your head in a plastic bag with a towel on top. Keep this on throughout the following.
**3.** Steam your face: add two drops of geranium oil to a bowl of just-boiled water. Put a large towel over your head and the bowl. Keep your face about 18 ins (45 cm) away from the water for about 10 minutes – but don't get uncomfortable. The steam opens and cleanses the pores. CAUTION: Do not steam if you have thread

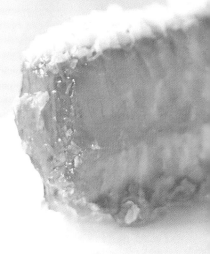

veins, are asthmatic, or suffer from a heart condition.

**4.** Make a cherry mask with fresh cherries. Crush them into a slushy paste and put all over your neck and face.

**5.** Run a hot bath. Add four drops of fennel oil to a cup of milk, mix and add to the bath. Soak for about 20 minutes. Drink a cup of green tea while in the bath.

**6.** Pat off the cherry mask. Finally, unwrap your hair and wash. Have another early night: beautiful dreams!

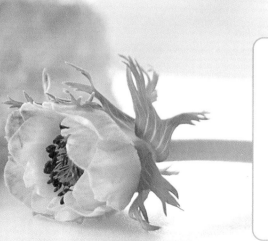

### RICH BODY CREAM

*15 ml beeswax*
*20 ml each almond and grapeseed oil*
*5 ml wheatgerm oil*
*20 ml rosewater or mineral water with*
 *5 drops of cider vinegar added*
*6 drops essential oil (either cypress,*
*fennel, juniper, mandarin, or neroli)*

*Melt the beeswax and pour into a small, heat-resistant bowl. Add the grapeseed, almond, and wheatgerm oils. Place the bowl in a pot of simmering water until the oils are blended and warm. Remove the bowl and slowly add the water – stir thoroughly all the time until the cream thickens and cools. Add your essential oil. Pour the cream into a sterilized jar. Refrigerate and use within a month.*

### LIGHT MOISTURIZER *(for most skins)*

*10 ml melted beeswax*
*45 ml wheatgerm oil*
*20 ml boiled water, mineral water, or rosewater*
*6 drops geranium oil (bergamot for oily skin)*

*Put the beeswax and oil in a small, heat-resistant bowl and place in a pot of boiling water. Stir thoroughly and remove the bowl from the pot. Slowly add the water, stirring all the time until the cream thickens and cools. Add the essential oil. Pour into a sterilized jar and refrigerate.*

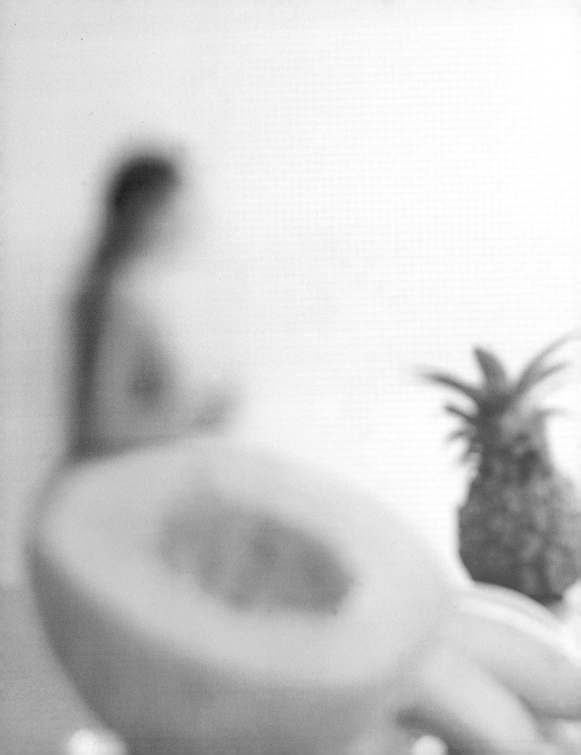

# Energizing weekend

*Energy is a vital commodity: if we could buy it, we'd all be racing to the store! Almost everyone complains that they don't have enough energy. It is not surprising as we are all living lives which are too busy, too stressful, too exhausting. When you feel in desperate of revitalizing, yourself try this weekend. It helps to restore your energy levels.*

**WHAT YOU'LL NEED:**
- *Food for energy (see page 41)*
- *Peppermint tea*
- *Essential oil: lavender*
- *Large sheets of paper, plus a set of crayons or paints*

# Friday evening RAISING ENERGY

This evening eat a light evening meal – maybe wholemeal
pasta with vegetable sauce and a little Parmesan cheese
sprinkled on top. Bring in energy-boosting food for the
weekend. Do some energy breathing and focus on colour
healing. Finally, get a good night's sleep after soaking in a
warm bath (add two or three drops of essential oil of
lavender) or ask someone to give you a gentle massage,
such as Ayurvedic abhyanga massage (see page 50).

## ENERGY BREATHING

This form of yogic breathing is called ujjayi, or the
"victorious" breath: it sends a balanced flow of energy
through both body and mind. Try ujjayi breathing several
times a day until you can do it at will.

**1.** Breathe in deeply, contracting the muscles around the
top of your windpipe. Pay attention to your throat and
you should hear a gentle hissing sound.

**2.** Breathe out as slowly as possible, closing off the
muscles around the epiglottis. Your breath rasps, as if
you were imitating Darth Vader from *Star Wars*.

**3.** Breathe in and out in this way six times.

**4.** Now relax and breathe normally.

**5.** If you have time, repeat this cycle (six ujjayi breaths
then six normal breaths) for four cycles.

## COLOUR HEALING

*If you constantly feel tired or under par, you may need a dose of red therapy!*

**1.** *Imagine the top of your head is opening and a beam of clear, red light is pouring down into you, filling up your body with healing energy.*

**2.** *While you visualize the colour, repeat to yourself "I bring into my body and mind all the energy I need". Keep going for around two minutes.*

**3.** *Now imagine the pores of your skin opening, so the light can filter through. As it escapes from your body, the light turns into a soft, pale mist that gently wraps itself around you, forming a cocoon of safety and healing.*

**4.** *You may feel a tingling of energy during this exercise. If you find it helps raise your energy levels, repeat daily.*

## THE ENERGY DIET

*Good food is the first step towards boosting energy. Follow these tips:*

✦ *Cut out sweets and sugar. They may provide an instant energy "high" but frequent consumption overstimulates insulin activity and leaves your energy depleted.*

✦ *Cut down on caffeine. Like sugar, it depletes the body's energy supplies.*

✦ *Eat plenty of complex carbohydrates, vegetables, and fruit (around 70% of your calorie intake); a much smaller amount of lean protein and some fat (from oily fish, olive oil, nuts). Avoid processed and refined foods, "junk" food, and pre-prepared meals see Energy Fish Dish page 152.*

✦ *Get enough vitamins and minerals – in particular B vitamins, chromium, and magnesium. Take good quality multi-vitamins and minerals plus additional antioxidants and the energy-boosting Co-enzyme Q10.*

# Saturday ENERGY FOR WELLBEING

Start the day with a salt massage bath (see page 35) but use cool water instead of warm. Enjoy a good breakfast. Try muesli (or porridge oats soaked overnight in soya milk). Add some dried fruits and nuts. Drink a glass of freshly squeezed orange juice and eat a couple of slices of wholemeal bread with honey.

Follow the steps of the Sun Salutation (see pages 148–149), a series of yoga moves which sends a surge of energy and wellbeing throughout your entire body (and mind!). Spend the rest of the morning decluttering and clearing your home (see page 76 for ideas). Clearing your home will enhance your energy levels enormously.

### ENERGY MUDRA

Eat scrambled eggs on wholemeal toast plus some fruit for lunch and then go for a brisk walk, breathing deeply (you can try the ujjayi energy breath while walking but you may need to slow down if you aren't used to it).

On your return, drink a cup of peppermint tea – it invigorates both body and mind. Then try the Apan Mudra – a yoga posture you do with your hands! It is also known as the Energy Mudra as it brings balance and calm, focused energy to you:

**1.** Place thumb, middle finger, and ring finger together and extend the other fingers. Do this with both hands.
**2.** Sit comfortably and rest your hands in this Mudra on your lap. Sit quietly for about 10 minutes or more.
**3.** Do this whenever you feel tired and in need of energy.

If possible, book yourself a massage this afternoon. Ideally, go for a dynamic form of bodywork, such as Indian rope massage (chavutti thirumal), shiatsu, tui na, or Thai massage. These all work on the inner energy systems of the body and will balance and re-energize your entire being.

## EVENING MEAL

In the evening, eat a light protein-packed meal of grilled tuna (or other fish see page 152) plus a salad.

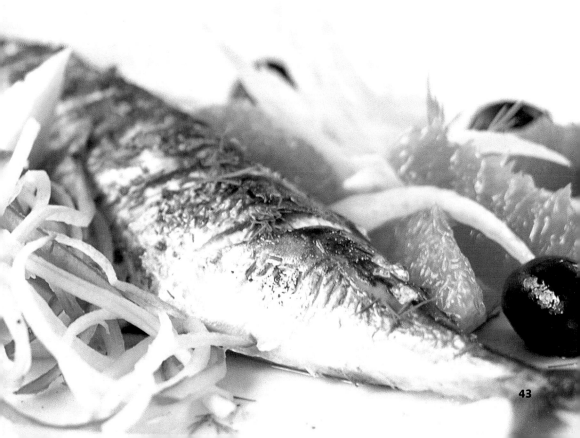

# Sunday BOOSTING YOUR ENERGY

Eat breakfast as for Saturday and afterwards experiment
with chi kung, the Chinese system of energy exercise.
Lunch is a baked potato filled with humus, fresh
tomatoes, and chopped onions plus a piece of fresh fruit.
Then go for a gentle walk (again try ujjayi energy
breathing). Dinner is Moroccan chicken (see page 152)
followed, after a rest, by the spinning exercise.

## STARTING POSITION OF CHI KUNG

The exercises look simple (and are) but they are
deceptively powerful. Use them whenever you need a
boost of focused energy. The following is the Starting
Position of chi kung. It puts you in the correct position
and helps you become aware of your entire body.
**1.** Stand with your feet shoulder-width apart. Find your
natural balance – if your weight is too far forward or too
far back it will cause tension and tiredness.
**2.** Feel the rim of your foot, your heel, your little toe, and
big toe relaxed on the ground.
**3.** Keep your knees relaxed. Check that your knees are
exactly over your feet.
**4.** Relax your lower back, stomach, and buttocks.
**5.** Let your chest become hollow. Relax and slightly
round your shoulders.
**6.** Imagine you have a pigtail on top of your head which
is tied to a rafter on the roof. Let your head float lightly
and freely. Relax your tongue, mouth and jaw.
**7.** Stay in this position for a few moments with your
hands hanging loosely by your sides.

## HOLDING THE DANTIEN

This exercise stimulates the Dantien, the storehouse of vital energy. The Dantien is located about two fingers' width below the navel.

**1.** Stand in the Starting Position.

**2.** Men should place their left hand on the Dantien, and the right hand over the left. Women should place their right hand on the Dantien with the left over it. Relax your whole body and lightly concentrate your thoughts on the Dantien.

**3.** With legs straight but not locked, breathe into the Dantien. Your abdomen will inflate under your hands.

**4.** Slowly bend your knees and breathe out. Your abdomen will deflate into the body on the out breath. Repeat this exercise for at least two minutes – as you get used to it, you can continue it for longer.

## THE SPINNING EXERCISE

The art and science of spinning is said to rejuvenate and energize your entire system. Simply stand erect with your arms outstretched, horizontal to the floor. Now, spin around clockwise, from left to right, until you feel slightly dizzy. Don't be surprised if you can only manage half a dozen spins to begin with – with time you will be able to build up your spinning.

Before you begin to spin, focus your vision on a single point straight ahead. As you begin to turn, hold your vision on that point for as long as possible and then refocus on the point as soon as possible.

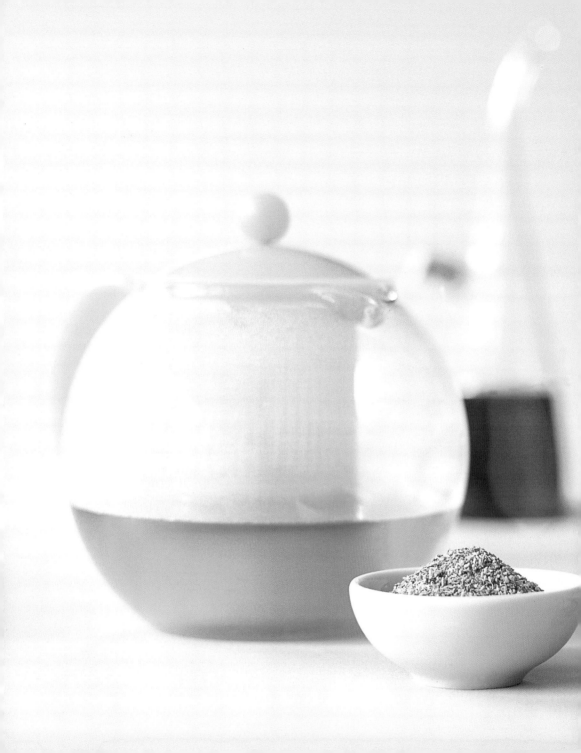

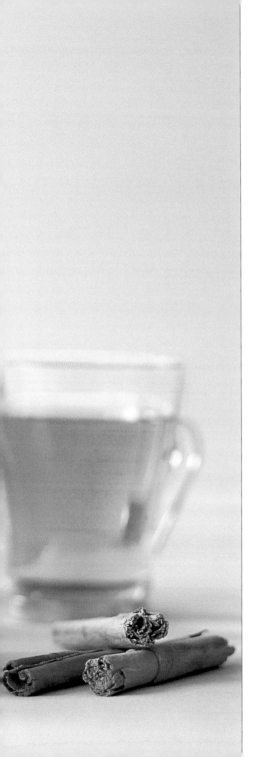

# Ayurveda weekend

*Ayurveda has been called the "Mother of Medicine" – with good cause. It is the ancient healing art of India, at least 5000 years old. What is most wonderful about Ayurveda is that it is a superb system of preventative medicine – it teaches us how to look after our bodies, minds, and souls, and bring them back to balance. This weekend should give you a taster.*

*WHAT YOU'LL NEED:*
- *Cold-pressed sesame oil*
- *Wholewheat chappatis*
- *Spicy or herbal teas (many health stores now stock Ayurvedic teas)*
- *Inspiring music and books*
- *"Garshan" glove or enough raw silk to make your own*

# Friday evening HEALING SOUNDS

Eat your evening meal no later than 6pm. The digestive fire, known in Ayurvedic medicine as agni, is at a low ebb by evening – so make this meal small and easily digested. Avoid heavy dairy produce, animal protein, and raw, cold foods at this meal.

   Go to bed early (no later than 10pm) – you will be having an early start!

## SINGING AND CHANTING

Think about introducing sound into your life – Ayurveda teaches that sound is one of the five subtle elements and can be very healing.

✦ The sounds of nature are soothing, balancing, and grounding. Spend some time outside and listen to birdsong, the hum of insects, or the wind in the trees.

✦ Make sounds yourself – singing (either full songs or sounds), toning, chanting, humming, groaning, shouting. These can all be therapeutic at differing times. Do you play an instrument? Would you like to learn? Which instrument would best suit you?

✦ Find a shop which specializes in "World Music" and ask for some advice on sacred Indian music.

✦ Some western Ayurvedic practitioners say that Gregorian chanting can be a good substitute for the classical Vedic music. You might like to investigate forms of overtone chanting from the Tibetan and Mongolian traditions as well, because these types of music appear to be deeply healing.

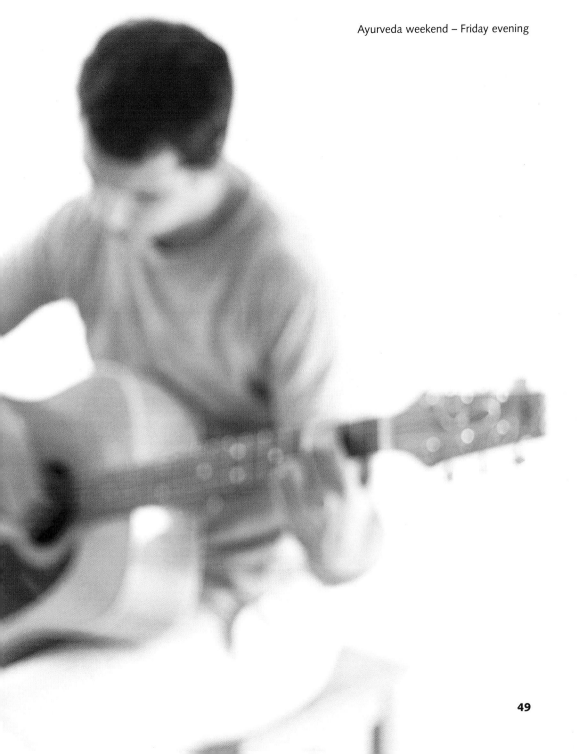

# Saturday GOOD DAILY ROUTINE

According to Ayurveda, a good daily routine is essential. What follows sounds stringent but do try to stick to it.

✦ Rise early – at sunrise or 5am (whichever is earlier). Urinate first thing after rising. If it's difficult, drink a glass of water or herbal tea (but not coffee).

✦ Brush your teeth, clean your tongue, gargle with cold water. Rinse your eyes with cool water. Trim your nails.

✦ Exercise: a long, fast walk, a swim, or yoga.

✦ Rub warm sesame oil into your body (don't worry too much about technique). Then take a body temperature bath to revitalize your body and stimulate your energy.

✦ Dress in loose, comfortable, clean clothing. Meditate, pray, or simply think about beautiful things.

✦ Now (at last) you can have breakfast. Eat it before 9am (no wonder you need an early start). Try dosas (see recipes on pages 152-53) – a classic Ayurvedic breakfast.

✦ Follow the breathing exercises on pages 19, 26, 40, and 87. Good breathing is an essential part of Ayurveda.

## THE LARGEST MEAL OF THE DAY

Lunch should be at least three hours later than breakfast – around one o'clock is fine. This should be the largest meal of the day as it's the time when your body can most easily digest food. Make dal with basmati rice (see recipes) and add some wholemeal chappatis if you are hungry. Go for a walk after your meal and then rest, listening to inspiring music.

## ABHYANGA MASSAGE

Mid-afternoon, when your meal is fully digested, you should have abhyanga, the basic Ayurvedic massage, in a warm, comfortable room. Try to arrange for someone to massage you – they don't need to be expert masseurs!

**1.** Lie naked on a large, warmed towel on the floor (this massage is very messy but you could wear an old pair of pants or a muslin loin cloth!) If you are massaging yourself it may be easier to sit upright.

**2.** Warm some cold-pressed sesame oil to body temperature (by placing in a bain-marie of hot water).

**3.** The abhyanga massage touch is light, rhythmic, and repetitive. Use circular movements over rounded areas, such as joints, and straight strokes over straight areas, such as the arms, legs, and neck.

**4.** Massage the oil gently into the scalp and neck.

**5.** Continue down the back and on to the hips and buttocks. Work down each leg in turn and pay particular attention to the feet (these can take a firmer pressure – make sure you massage between each toe).

**6.** Move back to the shoulders and work down each arm, making sure every inch is covered with oil – work down to the tip of each finger. Take your time – don't rush.

**7.** Turn over. Massage arms, legs, chest, and abdomen.

**8.** Finish with the neck and face. Gently massage every part of the face. Pull the ear lobes with a firm tug and massage inside the ear (don't poke – keep your fingers on the first ridge of the ear). Work gently inside each nostril.

**9.** Gently massage the third eye area (just between and above the eyebrows) with your thumb for five minutes.

**10.** Make sure you are warm (cover yourself with old towels or blankets) and relax for about 30 minutes.

**END OF THE DAY**
Eat a light meal (vegetable soup or a warm salad) before 6pm. Be in bed by 10pm, asleep before 11pm. If you're awake later it may be harder to get to sleep. Open a window in your bedroom – air should circulate freely.

# Sunday STIMULATE AND BALANCE

Follow the same routine as yesterday. But today, instead of abhyanga massage, you're going to use a technique called garshan, a highly stimulating treatment that boosts circulation, digestion, detoxification, and metabolism.

## GARSHAN MASSAGE

Unlike abhyanga, this massage is vigorous and uses a fair amount of pressure and quite a swift action. Wearing garshan gloves (see opposite) use long strokes over the large, long bones of the body and circular movements over the joints. Start by using 10 strokes per area – and gradually build up to around 40 or 50.

**1.** Start with the head, using circular movements, then stroke firmly down the neck and along the shoulder.

**2.** Use a circular motion over the shoulder joints then sweep with long strokes down the upper arms. Circle around the elbows and sweep down the forearms. Circle around the wrists and then finish up with long strokes over the hands and to the ends of the fingers.

**3.** Now move to the chest and use long strokes across the chest, from side to side, avoiding the area directly over the heart and breasts.

**4.** Move down to the abdomen and stroke from side to side, then diagonally across the abdomen. Work vigorously over the hips and buttocks.

**5.** Move down the legs – use long strokes down the thighs, circle over the knees, long strokes down the calves, circle around the ankles, and finish with long strokes down to the toes.

**GARSHAN GLOVES**

*Traditionally, garshan is performed with a pair of "gloves" made of raw silk, which is readily available from fabric shops. You can easily make a pair by drawing loosely around your hand to get the shape. Then sew the two pieces together with elastic around the wrist.*

## LUNCH

Eat lunch around 1pm – try spicy carrot and potato burgers with a side dressing of cucumber raita and a salad (but add something warm to it – such as croutons).

## AN AYURVEDIC EYE

This afternoon, look around your home with an Ayurvedic eye. You need a balance between the elements in your home. Think about incorporating the following:

✦ Earth: items of stone and terracotta; pebbles and sand; clay pots and vessels; large stones as doorstops; crystals.

✦ Water: bowls of water with petals floating on them or with pebbles at the bottom; water features such as fountains; fish tanks (with healthy fish).

✦ Air: open your windows at least once a day; burn incense and aromatherapy oils; turn on a fan.

✦ Fire: burn an open fire if you can, candles if you can't.

## END OF WEEKEND

Eat a light dinner at 6pm – soup or dhal and chappatis. Walk gently to aid digestion, then sit calmly and read for a while. Later, follow the Moon Salutation (pages 150–151). Afterwards, spend some time in quiet meditation or prayer. Be in bed by 10pm at the latest.

# Part two: mind and emotion

*Are you happy with the way you feel? Do you enjoy the way you spend your life – at work, at home, at play? Are your relationships warm and supportive, loving and exciting – or is love a battlefield? Do you feel fulfilled by your work or do you empathize with a hamster on its wheel, endlessly running in circles? Is your home a haven, a true sanctuary for the soul – a place in which you feel totally safe and secure? Or is it merely somewhere to hang your hat, a place to sleep and eat – and no more?*

*This part of the book looks at all these tough issues and offers suggestions to guide you to a happier, more harmonious life. Obviously you can't shift your entire mind and emotions in one weekend – it takes time and commitment. But you can surely set yourself on the right road.*

*Many of us don't even consider the subconscious – the great powerhouse of energy and creativity that lies beneath the conscious mind. The Explore your subconscious weekend can open up new avenues and prove a catalyst to deep and lasting change.*

*Break the Routine is ideal if you feel stuck in a rut – it's a great fun weekend and yet the simple shifts it suggests can have profound results. The Rearranging weekend takes a long hard look at all aspects of your life – from home to work to relationships – and suggests ways of instigating change.*

*Meanwhile, absolutely everyone in a relationship – whether you're in the first flush of romance or approaching your golden wedding anniversary – could derive great benefit from the Relationships weekend. It will help foster deeper understanding, intimacy – and introduce a large level of fun into your life.*

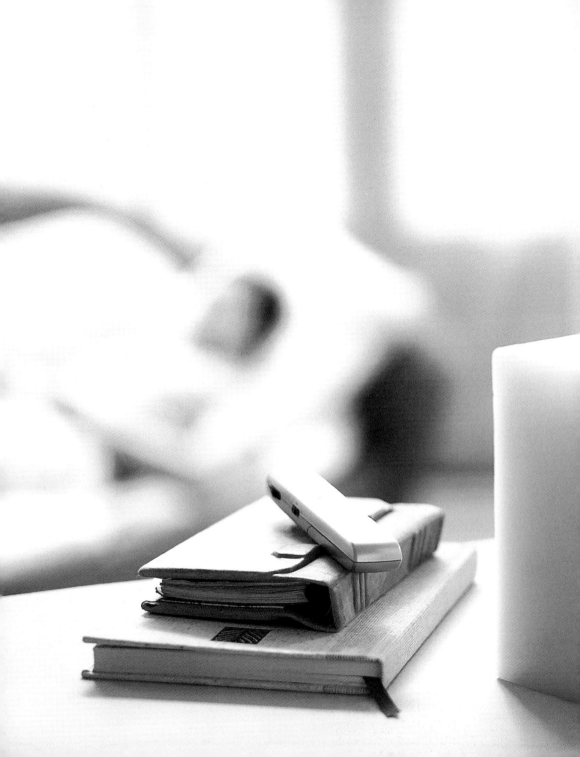

# Explore your subconscious

*Do you know who you are? You may think you do but you only use a fragment of your mind in everyday life. Beneath the surface lies a vast sea of the subconscious – a storehouse of vital information. Tap into it and let go of old fears, tame your demons, and unleash a flood of creativity and confidence.*

*CAUTION: some exercises in this weekend can work very deeply on the psyche. If you feel uncomfortable or scared at any point, you may need to consult a professional psychotherapist.*

*WHAT YOU'LL NEED:*
- *Essential oil: cedarwood (or helichrysum)*
- *Mugwort and scarlet monkeyflower flower essences (from the FES Quintessentials range)*
- *Tape recorder (optional)*
- *Paper, crayons, and paints*
- *Journal and pens*
- *Candles (purple or blue)*

# Friday evening GOING BACK IN TIME

Eat a light meal and then try the movement and art exercises from the Body Awareness weekend (see pages 14–21). These should start to free up your psyche. Write down any thoughts or images that emerge. Then do the guided visualization below.

Afterwards, enjoy a long, relaxing bath (add 4 drops of cedarwood – or, if you can get it, helichrysum – oil in a little milk). Don't be tempted to read a book before or in bed. Spend 10 to 20 minutes in quiet meditation (gently gaze at a candle flame). Reflect on any image or phrase that came up in the movement exercise or while bathing.

Take a drop of mugwort flower essence on your tongue before sleep to help you remember your dreams. Keep your journal and a pen by your bed – or a tape recorder – to capture your dreams if you wake in the night.

## GUIDED VISUALIZATION

This exercise can take you back in time to uncover repressed or forgotten material. Do it with a friend if you can. You may wish to tape record your comments. If you are on your own, tape the following instructions and leave plenty of pauses in between each step so you can relax totally and work with your experience.

CAUTION: If you know (or have suspicions) that you were abused then I would advise you to work with a qualified psychotherapist or hypnotherapist rather than do this exercise on your own.

**1.** Sit or lie somewhere comfortable and warm. Gently close your eyes. Check your body is relaxed (run through each part of your body tensing and relaxing it in turn).

**2.** Spend a few minutes just becoming aware of your breathing – it gets slower and deeper as you relax.

**3.** Tell yourself that it's safe to let yourself go deeper and

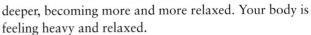

deeper, becoming more and more relaxed. Your body is feeling heavy and relaxed.

**4.** Any troubling thoughts are like ripples on a pond: you watch them as they slowly move out and away, leaving the pond clear and perlucid.

**5.** Any remaining thoughts are like clouds in the sky. You watch them flurry away, leaving the sky clear and blue.

**6.** Now imagine you are standing at the top of a series of 10 steps. Slowly you walk down the steps. As you place your foot on each step you feel yourself becoming more relaxed, more deeply relaxed, going deeper down. Count from one to 10 slowly, knowing that each step is taking you further back in time.

**7.** When you reach 10, you are totally relaxed, totally calm. Before you is a door. When you open the door, you will be at a time in the past which is meaningful to you.

**8.** Open the door and step through.

**9.** Look down at your feet. Are they smaller? What are you wearing on them?

**10.** Look at your hands and any other parts you can see.

**11.** Now slowly start to look around you. Where are you? Who's with you? What is happening?

**12.** Just follow what happens.

**13.** When you're ready (you can leave at any time), walk back to and through the door. Walk slowly up the steps, counting from 10 to one. As you walk on each step you become more aware, more awake, more conscious of your body lying on the floor or sitting in a chair.

**14.** When you reach the top you are fully awake, fully aware. Slowly open your eyes, slowly get up and stamp your feet. Drink a glass of water and eat something (to ground you solidly back in the present).

**15.** Write down your experiences in your journal.

# Saturday INTO THE LIGHT OF DAY

Immediately you wake up, lie still and recall any dreams you have had. Write them down, or record them on tape, as soon as you have remembered them.

Today you're going to bring some of what you've found into the light of day – through bodywork, art therapy, and free association.

This morning, attend a session of bodywork. Our emotions aren't held just in our heads, but in our muscles, tendons, and even our bones. A good bodyworker can help release old memories and let you discover the basis of old patterns of behaviour. The most effective systems include SHEN®, biodynamic massage, Rolfing, Hellerwork, myofascial massage, and watsu (a combination of shiatsu and water therapy) – but any form of bodywork will be useful.

Afterwards write down any thoughts, images, and emotions that emerged.

## ART THERAPY

Get out your paints – it's time for some art therapy. Find a space where you can paint freely. You need to be able to pin up some large sheets of paper (newspaper will do) and make a mess. Kitchens can usually be easily cleaned (or maybe the bathroom if it's big enough!). A garage is another option. Wear old clothes, too – you need to be totally uninhibited.

Turn to page 94 and follow the guidelines. When you feel you've finished, sit back and look at your paintings. What are they saying to you? What images can you see in the paint? Let your imagination hold sway. If your painting could talk, what would it say? Write down your thoughts in your journal.

## FREE ASSOCIATION

This evening, make time for breathing and yoga (see Part One's weekends for ideas). These practices will help you to process the subconscious material that's emerging.

If you feel you're progressing well with the painting, you could continue it this evening, perhaps by candlelight or while listening to music.

If you would prefer a change, try free association. Light a blue or purple candle and sit down with your journal (or a pad of paper) and pen. Write whatever comes into your head – however silly or meaningless. Don't censor yourself in any way. You might write the same thing over and over for pages – just trust in the process. If you find it hard to start then try one of these phrases:

✦ "I want......"
✦ "I hate......."
✦ "If I'm really honest...."
✦ "I wish I could......"

If you find yourself getting into difficult emotions, pause and take a few deep breaths.

Afterwards take the same bath as you enjoyed on Friday (see page 58).

# Sunday FACING YOUR SHADOW

What did you dream last night? Your activities over the weekend so far should have thrown up some interesting dreams. Record them as you did yesterday.

Then get some exercise! Go for a long walk, or a swim, or a session at the gym. Or do some yoga, Pilates, or stretching. Whatever you do, get your body moving. You could always put on loose clothes and dance at home.

✦ Spend some time connecting with your breath.

✦ What does your body want to do? Just let your body move in whatever way it wishes. It might want to stomp around the room like a five year old or swoop like a bird.

✦ Do you need music? Possibly not. But if you do, what kind of music does your body want? Follow its lead.

## SHADOW FIGURES

We're going to get in touch with our shadows. In Jungian psychology the shadow is the part of us that contains all the behaviour, thoughts, and emotions that we hide away from conscious life. If you ever have dreams with a frightening figure of the same sex as yourself (the murderer, overbearing teacher, the harlot, the bully) or someone despicable and horrible (the wimp, the whining child, the dirty tramp) you have met your shadow. Anything we can't cope with in our own psyches, we push away and it becomes our shadow.

If you ignore the shadow, it can fester and grow. Sometimes it can break out in a worrying way – such as when we get blind drunk and violent; or lash out in fury; or find ourselves in bed with someone we don't even like!

The ideal solution is not to destroy or dismiss the shadow; but to integrate it into our conscious life. The shadow contains huge reservoirs of energy that we can use – positively.

## SHADOW WORK

Before you start these exercises, take a couple of drops of scarlet monkeyflower flower essence to help put you in touch with your shadow.

**1.** List everyone who really annoys or irritates you – from people you know well to celebrities or even soap stars.

**2.** Why do you dislike them? Which characteristics really bug you?

**3.** Are there any groups of people you find frightening or unpleasant? Be honest. Behind a lot of racism, for example, is deep shadow work.

**4.** Now think about these qualities. Do you possess them within you? Or have you denied them in yourself? If you aren't ready to take this step of owning your shadow, don't worry: you have done valuable groundwork.

**5.** Try painting your shadow. Although quite frightening at first, remember a painting is a safe container for your fears. If it still feels threatening, paint a big frame around the picture to contain it while you work with it.

**6.** Use the "other chair" technique (see page 86). Put your shadow in one chair, you in the other.

**7.** Write to your shadow. What would you tell it?

8. Watch out for shadow figures in your dreams. Work in this way with any such figures: i.e. paint them, talk with them, write to them, communicate with them.

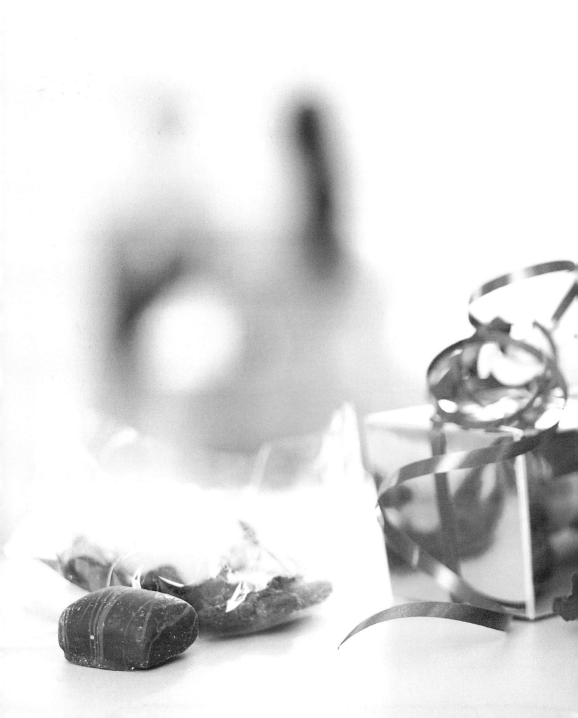

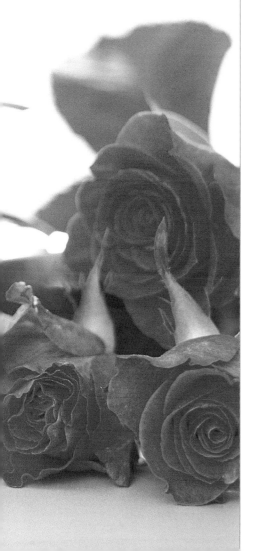

# Relationships weekend

*If our relationships were plants they would probably have withered and died years ago! We neglect our nearest and dearest in the most appalling ways. This weekend is planned to nourish and support every partnership: if your relationship is new it will help you get to know each other better; if you have been together a long time it will help rekindle the early sparkle.*

*WHAT YOU'LL NEED:*
- *Favourite foods*
- *Essential oils: geranium, and your choice of ylang ylang or sandalwood*
- *Sweet almond oil*
- *Candles: one red, one pink, one yellow*
- *Paper and pens*

# Friday evening CLOSENESS AND TRUST

Prepare and cook a meal together and maybe buy a bottle of wine to share (but don't get drunk!). While you're eating, reminisce on how you met. What were your first impressions? What did you say and do? Was it instant attraction or a slower burn? Recall your early dates: when you first kissed; when you first slept together.

After you have finished eating, sit down comfortably and try this exercise:

**1.** Take half an hour each to talk about how you feel and what you want in life – as if you were explaining yourself to a stranger. While each person talks, the other must be silent and listen with full attention.

**2.** After half an hour change roles.

**3.** At the end of the hour stop the conversation and don't dissect it. Wait until Sunday to revisit the discussion.

## YOGA FOR INTIMACY

Yoga is a wonderful way of fostering closeness, trust, and understanding – in fact, the word yoga actually means "union". Practising yoga with your partner can really help you connect. The following poses are especially designed to be performed in pairs.

Set aside plenty of time for this exercise. Be aware of any feelings that come up – either in your body or in your mind and emotions. Take time after your practice to talk about what it felt like for you both.

## BREATHING TOGETHER

**1.** Sit back to back on the floor, with legs crossed. Shift your buttocks so you are nestling close to each other, fully supporting each other. Lean back into your partner.

**2.** Become aware of your partner's back. Where are you touching? Feel the breath in your back.

## THE TWIST

**1.** Sit cross-legged on the floor, facing each other. Keep your back straight yet relaxed. Move your knees as close as you can to your partner's.

**2.** Gaze into each other's eyes and breathe together deeply three times.

**3.** Now you both place the back of your left hand against your lower back, a few inches above your tailbone.

**4.** Both of you twist towards the left, reaching your right hand past the left side of your partner's body to clasp the hand behind your partner's back. Turn your heads and look over your left shoulder, away from each other.

**5.** Hold this stretch (you may want to lean back a little further from each other to intensify the stretch).

**6.** Take a deep breath and twist further as you exhale. Breathe deeply in this position for five deep breaths.

**7.** Unclasp your hands and bring them back to your lap. Turn to face your partner.

**8.** Repeat steps 3 to 6 on the other side.

## THE SEESAW

**1.** Sit on the floor facing each other. Spread your legs out as far as is comfortable and touch your toes together.

**2.** Reach forwards and clasp each other around the elbows (or wrists or hands).

**3.** Gently gaze into each other's eyes and begin to rock gently backwards and forwards (as if you were rowing).

**4.** Try to breathe in synchronization with your partner. Try to find a rhythm which suits you both.

**5.** Complete 10 stretches and then return to the central position. Gently close your eyes and hold hands. Just sit quietly for a few minutes.

# Saturday OPENNESS AND HONESTY

Start the day with a cuddle. Just lie in bed and hold each other for a few minutes (or as long as you like!). When you eat breakfast (either in bed or out of the house), each of you should make a list of 10 things you'd love to do as a couple (don't let the other see until you've finished).

First one then the other intuitively picks an activity on their list – and then you do it together! If one of you really hates the other's choice then try to be open and enthusiastic. Recognize this is something your partner wants to do – so give it a go (you might even enjoy it!).

## SEX LIVES

This evening cook another light meal together. As you chop and stir, imagine you're putting the love, intimacy, and fun you want for your relationship in the pan.

Sex is an important part of relationships but it's an area we often leave to luck. Few couples actually talk honestly

---

**GOOD COMMUNICATION**
*Avoid misunderstandings with these ground rules:*
✦ *Make sure you're both calm when you talk.*
✦ *Talk in terms of feelings and thoughts – i.e. "I feel [upset, hurt, angry, insecure, etc.] about [specific action or statement by your partner]" – rather than "You are a mean, selfish bastard" or similar.*
✦ *Be specific, never general.*
✦ *Say what you really mean rather than speaking in code, i.e. instead of "Your friend Bob drinks too much" tell the truth – you're upset your partner is spending more time with Bob than with you.*
✦ *Suggest practical, specific solutions where possible, i.e. "How would it be if you saw Bob and your work friends on Fridays while we go out on Thursdays?"*

---

and candidly about what works and what doesn't in their sex lives. Sex therapists say that honest communication can transform sex. Ask each other the following:
+ Am I doing to you what you'd like me to do?
+ What might we like if only we tried?
   Sit down and talk about it calmly. How often would you like to make love? What would make it better for you? What are your fantasies? You may be surprised.

## LOVING MASSAGE
Give each other a massage this evening – touching in a loving, caring way deeply nourishes any relationship.
**1.** Warm the room and place towels on the floor.
**2.** Light three candles – pink for romance, yellow for friendship, and red for passion. Put a few drops of sandalwood or ylang ylang essential oils in a burner.
**3.** Make up a massage oil by mixing 6 drops of either oil in four teaspoons (20 ml) of sweet almond oil.
**4.** Start by massaging your partner's back – use a circular movement (up either side of the spine and then swooping around the outer edges of the back). Check with your partner that you are using the right amount of pressure.
**5.** Squeeze and press the tight muscles around the neck and shoulders.
**6.** Knead any fleshy areas – such as hips and thighs.
**7.** Try other techniques: turn your hands into fists and (with fingers against the skin) gently pummel; cup your hands and move over the skin as if you were drumming.
**8.** Make small, circling movements over the shoulders, the soles of the feet, palms of the hands, and the chest. Use long, stroking movements down the arms and legs.
**9.** Be inventive – let your hands guide you and remember you can't get it wrong if your partner is enjoying it!

# Sunday STRENGTHENING THE BOND

Share an invigorating shower together – use a few drops
of geranium oil to make you feel cheered and optimistic.
Then choose another activity from your love-to-do lists.

## AFTERNOON PLAYTIME
Researchers have found that a sense of fun and play
helps couples communicate better, strengthens their
bond, and helps prevent conflict. Married couples who
lose their sense of play find their relationship rapidly
deteriorates. So have fun together this afternoon:
◆ Share childhood stories. Get out old photo albums and
really reminisce.
◆ Find out what your partner's favourite toy or game
was as a child and buy him or her one as a present.
◆ Watch a favourite movie, cartoon, or old TV show on
video. Stock up on choc ices, popcorn, and indulge!
◆ Role play one of your favourite movie scenes – let your
imagination run wild.

## REVISITING FRIDAY EVENING
If one of you always does the cooking, it's time for the
non-cook to take over the pans. Try to cook a meal that
you know your partner will really enjoy (see page 152).
If you never usually cook, don't be too ambitious – but
do make an effort (rather than just sending out for food
or microwaving a ready meal!).

  After dinner sit down together – you might burn some
geranium oil and light the candles again. Discuss the
conversation you had on Friday. Take it in turns to talk
and be honest.

If you find it hard to get started, try asking yourselves these questions:

**1.** If you have decisions to make or problems to solve does it ever feel as if you are on opposing teams?

**2.** Do you ever argue about money?

**3.** Do you tend to change the subject if a difficult topic (sex, commitment, money, parents, children) comes up?

**4.** Can you reveal things to each other that might be humiliating or really embarrassing?

**5.** If you wanted a really fun day out would you tend to turn to your friends rather than your partner?

**6.** What works in your relationship? What doesn't?

**7.** Does your partner ever do/say things that make you irritated or uncomfortable?

**8.** Do either of you hold ideas or cherish plans that would make your relationship difficult to continue?

**9.** What have you learned about your partner this weekend?

**10.** Can you imagine yourselves happily together in 10 years' time?

You can either swap answers or use them as a basis for frank discussion.

**KEEP PLAYING**

*This evening, in bed, play games and tell each other stories…take it in turns to tell ghost stories (with the lights off); do puppet shows with your hands and a torch; trace shapes on your partner's back with your finger and have him/her guess what you've drawn.*

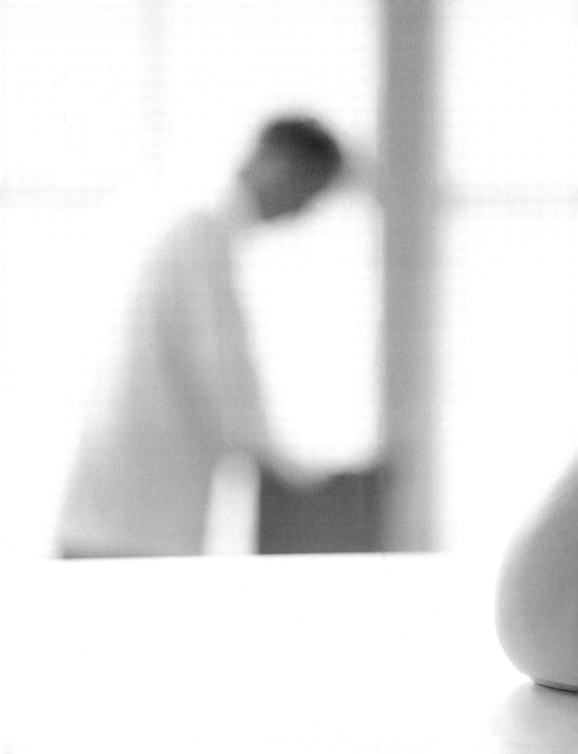

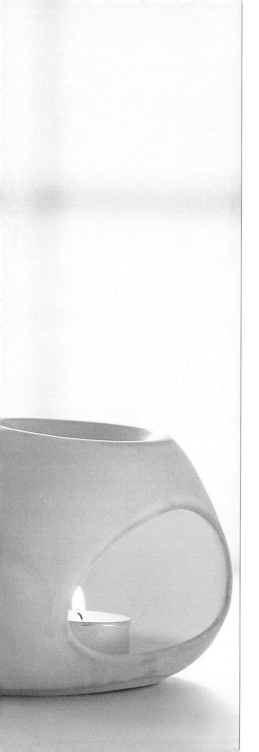

# Rearranging weekend

*Do you like your life? Are you happy with your home, your work, your relationships? Or do they need a little rearranging, some genuine decluttering? If you feel that your life needs some tweaking so you can function at your best, then try this weekend: it should blow away your cobwebs and freshen up some parts of your life.*

*WHAT YOU'LL NEED:*
- *Candle (either red, yellow, or green)*
- *Aromatherapy burner and oils (juniper or lemon)*
- *Paper and coloured pens*
- *Large bags and/or boxes*

# Friday evening LOOKING AT YOUR LIFE

Light a candle (yellow for optimism, red for dynamism, or green for balance and fresh starts). Burn a little lemon or juniper oil to uplift and cheer you. Get a large bottle of water or pour a glass of wine! Write the following headings and answer the questions in a list on separate sheets of paper:

◆ Work: what do you do (be precise)? Who do you see (on a daily and more occasional basis)? Where do you go for work (do you stay in one place or move around)?

◆ Home: where do you live? What do you do at home (what activities)? How much time do you spend there? Who do you see (people living with you or visitors)?

◆ Family: who's in your family (who lives with you and who doesn't)? What do you do together?

◆ Friends: who are they? What do you do with them?

◆ Hobbies: what are your hobbies? When, where, and with whom do you do them?

◆ Spirituality: what are your beliefs? Do you go to a place of worship? Do you meditate or pray?

Underline the parts of your lists that work really well with a green pen; all the parts that are bearable with an orange pen; and the bits that really don't work for you with a red pen. Be brutally honest – nobody needs to see this but you. You may be surprised at the results – often it's not the whole situation (i.e. work) that we hate; but just elements of it.

Place your lists under your pillow at night. Let your unconscious mind come up with some good solutions while you sleep. Keep a pad and pen by your bed – inspiration can come through dreams and you'll need to jot it down before you forget it.

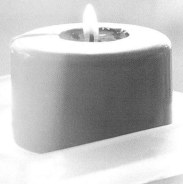

## ASK THE MIRACLE QUESTION

If don't have enough time this evening for this solution-focused therapy then try it at another point in the weekend. Sit down and ask yourself the following questions (or have someone else ask you):

**1.** If, when you woke up, your problems had vanished, how would you know a miracle had happened? If your reaction is to say something like "I wouldn't be depressed any more" or "I would discover I'd won the lottery" try going beyond and looking at how you would feel.

**2.** How would you behave differently (be precise)?

**3.** How would your family or friends behave differently?

**4.** How would they know a miracle had happened? How would they see the differences in your behaviour?

**5.** What parts of the miracle are already happening?

**6.** How have you made them happen? Can you get more of them to happen?

**7.** What in your present life would you like to continue?

**8.** On a scale of 0 to 10 (where 0 is the worst your life has been and 10 is the day after the miracle) where are you now?

**9.** If you are on, say, four, how would you get to five? What would you be doing differently?

**10.** How would your family and friends know you had moved up a point?

These questions sound simple but they are focusing on your thoughts and behaviour – something you have the power to change. For example, if you said you were no longer depressed you might be more relaxed, happier, more peaceful. How would your family know? You might play with the children more; call up your parents to chat; get up earlier. Those are all things you can alter if you choose.

# Saturday THE BIG CLEAR OUT

Jot down any thoughts that you may have had in the
night (if you haven't had any, don't worry!). This
morning you're going to start decluttering and sorting
out your house! You probably won't get it completed
over the weekend so set aside an hour or so each week.

Eat a swift, light breakfast (maybe a fruit smoothie or
some fruit salad and muesli) first. Wear old clothes and
get several large bin bags (or boxes) to hand. Put on some
music and burn juniper or lemon oil to give you a helpful
push. Be ruthless.

✦ Throw out old medicines, cosmetics, and food –
they're all bad for you.

✦ Thin out your books and music collection – you can
always get hold of them again if you really need them.

✦ Recycle newspapers and magazines – cut out the bits
you really want and put in a neat file or stick in a book.

✦ Donate old, unwanted clothes, ornaments, or nick-
nacks to charity. If it's a family "heirloom" offer it to
other family members. If they don't want it – sell it!

## THE RIGHT EXERCISE

Eat a good, healthy lunch. Get some exercise this
afternoon but check you're not wasting time on the
wrong sort. Do you enjoy your exercise? If not, what
would you like to do?

Think about what you want to achieve from your
workout. What's the point of running for hours if all you
want are trim arms? For weight loss pick high-intensity
sports such as running, stair climbing, aerobics, and fast
cycling coupled with strength-work. For stress relief pick
yoga, tai chi, or boxing. If you simply want to improve
your overall fitness level then opt for low impact
aerobics, swimming, and walking.

## MAKE CHANGES THAT SUPPORT YOU

Cook yourself a comforting 'soul' supper of soup and wholemeal bread plus a vitamin-packed fruit salad. Now take out your pens again and find a comfortable corner.

Look through your list from last night. How could you make changes that would support you? For example, do you really love your hobbies? Are you learning a new language because you adore it or because it's an impressive dinner party topic? Do you cook gourmet food when you'd rather be watching a video and eating a take-out? Only do what you really enjoy or really need.

Are you still seeing people who bore you rigid or are you frustrated because you don't have the time to see the people who are important to you? Be brutal (but not cruel) and lose a few pages from your address book.

If time is a problem, become proactive. Decide who to see and when. Plan what to do and when. Block off time in your diary for friends, exercise, and hobbies and treat them just like real appointments with someone else, only breaking them if absolutely unavoidable.

You should find many areas resolve themselves but, if you have any sticky ones, place your list under your pillow again and ask your subconscious for guidance.

# Sunday MAXIMIZING ENERGY

This morning you will be rearranging your home to
maximize its energy, or chi, according to feng shui, the
Chinese art and science of energy placement.

◆ Walk through your home as if you were seeing it and
sensing it for the very first time. What impression do you
get? Which rooms "work" and which don't feel right?

◆ Do a clutter check. Clutter drags down your energy
so do some more (brutal) clearing.

◆ Energy enters through your front door. Make sure it
is welcoming and opens, if possible, into a spacious and
well-lighted interior. The door should open inwards so
the energy enters smoothly. Make sure all the lights are
working and that the hallway is bright and welcoming.

◆ Avoid long corridors. If a corridor ends with a blank
wall put a mirror there. Break up a row of doors with a
crystal or a wind-chime.

◆ Energy should move slowly and smoothly but its flow
can easily be blocked by too many obstacles in its path.
So avoid protruding furniture in corridors and sharp
corners. When chi is blocked the effect is usually felt in
the residents' marriages and financial affairs. Put up
mirrors to smooth over tight corners.

◆ Energy stagnates in perpetually dark or unused places.
Rooms should be well lighted and well used. Keep rooms
that are seldom used clean and free from dust.

◆ Energy flows well in sunlight. Keep your home as light
and bright as possible.

◆ Healthy energy is attracted by life, movement, and
sound. Hang wind chimes which tinkle in the breeze;
place healthy live plants throughout; keep fish in
bubbling aquaria or install a water fountain.

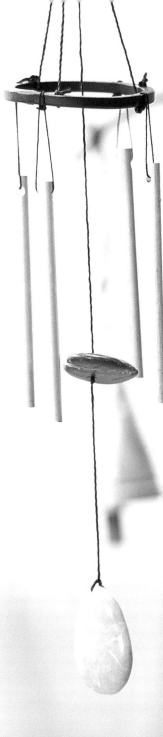

## THE CORE STATEMENT

Work is often a sticking point. We need to work (well, most of us do) but it makes many of us unhappy. If this weekend's exercises have made you wonder about your work, try this technique, called the Core Statement. It helps you discover what would really "make your soul sing". You might find that all you need to do is to shift your focus like the salesman who was energized by the risk of having no fixed income – once he went on to a safe salary he became unhappy.

If you can, ask another person to write down any phrases or words which you emphasize or repeat. If you're working alone, tape it.

**1.** Find a joyful childhood memory. What were you doing? What made it special? How did you feel? Was anyone with you? Which aspect did you enjoy the most? Write down the key phrases and words which occur.

**2.** Think of a good time in your life – at any period. Ask the same questions as before and again write down the key phrases and words.

**3.** Repeat the above process with the following: a hobby or pastime; a fulfilling work experience; and a moment when you felt complete.

**4.** Write the most important key phrases and words on a piece of paper. Which keep occurring? Where are the patterns? Which represent the most important circumstances or attitudes? If you could only have three or four of these phrases or words, which would they be?

**5.** Try to put them together in a sentence with real meaning for you. When you hit on the right kind of statement it will instinctively feel right – some people laugh or even cry. Play with it until it works for you.

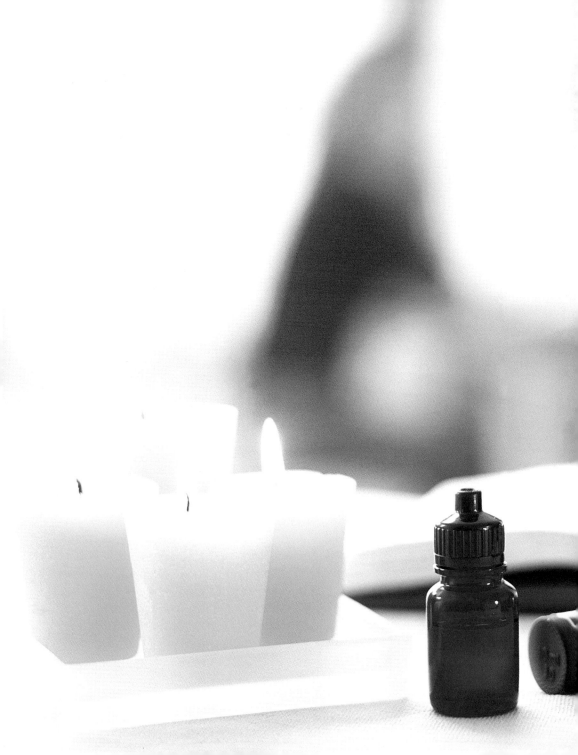

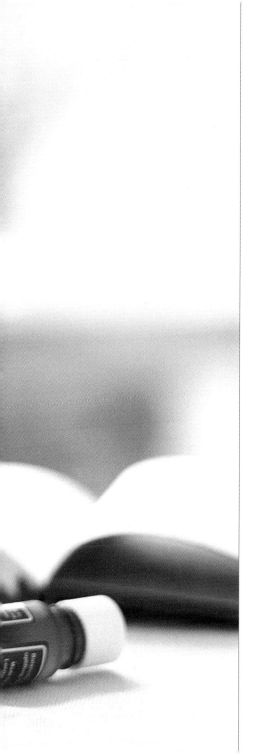

# Break your routine

*Sometimes you look at your life and realize you're stuck in a rut. You've been following the same routine day in, day out for a long while and are feeling jaded and bored. So it's time to jolt yourself into a whole new lifestyle. Obviously you can't change your entire life in a weekend, but you can make a good start. At the very least this weekend will start to challenge your perceptions and shift your consciousness into a brand-new pattern.*

*WHAT YOU'LL NEED:*
- *Food and drink – a selection that is completely different from usual*
- *Essential oils: pine or lemon*
- *Green candle*
- *Pen and paper, crayons or paints*
- *Walnut Bach flower remedy*

# Friday evening FRESH BEGINNINGS

Tonight you're going to be doing a fair amount of writing
and thinking so choose a meal that is easy to prepare.
Which of the following would you never normally eat?
Fish and chips; Indian or Chinese to go; a humus
sandwich; miso soup; tofu stirfry? Choose one which you
have never (or rarely) eaten before.

## THINKING ABOUT ROUTINE

**1.** Light a green candle (to symbolize fresh beginnings)
and maybe burn pine or lemon aromatherapy oil.

**2.** Write down how you spend your life now. What is
your daily routine? Be specific: do you always get up in
the same way? What do you eat for breakfast? How do
you get to work, etc?

**3.** Do you do specific things on specific days? Do you
take your holidays at the same time or go to the same
place? How much routine is there in your life?

**4.** How does this make you feel? Do you feel comforted
by routine or stifled by it? Sometimes it's hard to tell until
you try making a shift. This weekend you are going to do
things completely differently, as often as possible. It may
sound contrived but just try it. Sometimes even a small or
silly shift can produce a radically different perspective
and open up new opportunities. So play with this.

**5.** Next to every entry on your paper, write down
something opposite or totally different. For instance: buy
a croissant on the way to work for breakfast: make a
home breakfast of fresh fruit salad and muesli.

**6.** Go through the day in this way and resolve to shift
absolutely everything you can this weekend.

## WISHFUL THINKING

Take out a large sheet of paper and make a list of 100 things you really wish you could do in your life. They don't need to be practical or sensible and they can range from the small and humdrum (get a haircut; buy some incense) to the medium range (visit a health farm; learn to read the Tarot; go to French evening classes) to really wild scenarios (start your own business; travel round the world; have cosmetic surgery; move to another country).

At the end of the weekend commit yourself to doing at least one during the following week. Underline what you would really love to do. Make a time frame: commit to doing some in the next year. Work out what you could do towards achieving your long-term goals – for example, put aside a small amount of money each week towards that round-the-world trip; find out how to re-train for your ideal career; spend an hour each day (or week) writing your novel.

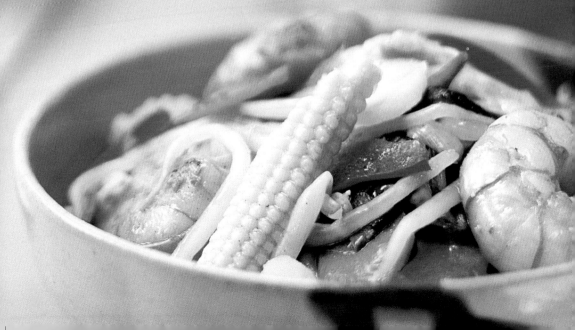

# Saturday NEW PERSPECTIVES

Before you get up, shift your morning regime. If you're usually up at the crack of dawn, try lying in bed, just thinking or with a book. How does it feel to relax like this? If you are a habitual lie-in-bed, set your alarm for dawn and get up with the birds. Prepare to spend the day shifting your perspectives and breaking habits.

Get out and about, trying new things. Be spontaneous. If you usually drive, take a bus, train, or taxi. Don't grab that usual sandwich, treat yourself in a smart restaurant. If you often eat alone, arrange to meet a friend. Then go to at least three shops you would never normally visit. Keep an open mind. In the evening do something you would never usually do: a classical concert, a rock gig; go salsa dancing or take a walk in the moonlight. Stay in and pamper yourself (see Beauty weekend for ideas); turn off the television (or, if you never watch it, turn it on!). Whatever you do, make sure it is different.

## BALANCING YOUR WOOD ELEMENT
According to Chinese philosophy, the body is a blend of five elements. The Wood element relates to creativity and expression and if Wood is balanced in your body you will be far more flexible and creative, confident and decisive. Help bring Wood into balance with these simple shiatsu and stretching exercises:

**1.** Sit on the floor with your legs spread wide apart. Reach down to your left foot, looking at your right foot, feeling the full stretch down your side and legs. Repeat on the other side.

**2.** Stand up with your feet apart. Let your arms swing loosely from side to side for a few minutes. Feel the air on your arms. Be as loose and relaxed as possible.

**3.** Lie on your back. Let a friend or partner rotate the

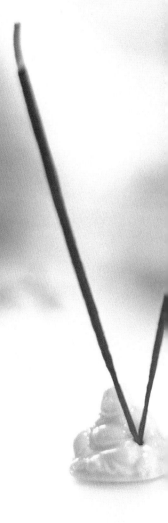

joints of your shoulders and hips. Gently and smoothly they should lift your leg or arm and support the shoulder or hip with the other hand. If the joint sticks, gently pull the limb and hold the stretch for a few moments. It should feel good, not painful – don't go beyond what feels comfortable.

**4.** Further stimulate the Wood element in your body with yoga or by following a full series of stretches every day. Try the Sun and Moon Salutations on pages 148–151.

## FEEL A STONE'S ENERGY

Go out to your garden, a park, or wild place nearby. Look for a stone, one that "speaks to you". You'll know it when you find it. Pick it up and sit quietly with it (or sit by it if it's a huge boulder!). Feel it (with your fingers and hands, against your face); smell it; look at it closely; taste it. Get to know it really well. Now imagine you actually ARE that stone. What is it like? Feel the stone's energy. Don't race this exercise – stone energy is not a swift thing, it takes time and patience.

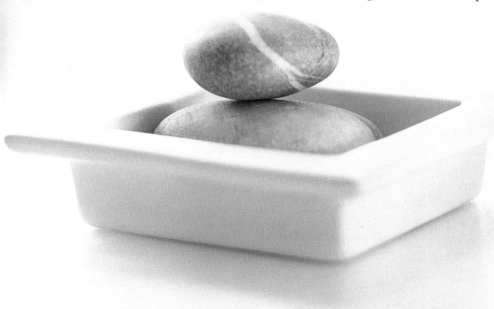

# Sunday SEEING THE WORLD DIFFERENTLY

What kind of spiritual life do you have? Do you have any spiritual practice? This morning think about expanding your spiritual perspective. Are you a regular worshipper? Think about visiting another place of worship, either of your own or a different faith. Or stay at home and spend some time in meditation and quiet prayer.

If you have no faith and no spiritual practice, think about your relationship to the divine. If you have a longstanding dislike of church or synagogue or mosque, maybe now is the time to re-evaluate. If there is a service this morning, why not go? If not, maybe just visit to get a feel for the place.

## TRANSFORM A DIFFICULT RELATIONSHIP

We can get into bad habits with people just as easily as we can with our activities. This afternoon try a technique to break such a habit. Think of someone with whom you have a bad or difficult relationship?

**1.** Sit or lie down and breathe calmly and deeply.

**2.** Write down your reasons for the bad relationship. Pour out all your resentment and any feelings of anger.

**3.** Set up two chairs. Sit in one and imagine the other person is sitting in the other. Tell them exactly why you find them so difficult.

**4.** Swap chairs and imagine you are the other person. Why do they find you so difficult or unreasonable? Slip into their shoes and express their grievances.

**5.** Swap chairs like this until you understand both sides of the issue. Try to accept that there are two sides to every disagreement. People are just different!

**6.** Burn the piece of paper containing your grievances.

**7.** Send unconditional love to the person. This may be hard but persist as it is deeply transformative.

## BRAIN GYM
Belly breathing and brain buttons are Educational Kinesiology exercises which will help you re-tune your brain and start seeing the world in a different way.

## BRAIN BUTTONS
This stimulates the carotid arteries which supply freshly oxygenated blood to the brain. It helps re-establish directional messages from parts of the body to the brain, so improving reading, writing, speaking, and the ability to follow directions.

**1.** Rest one hand over your navel.

**2.** With the thumb and fingers of the other hand, feel for the two hollow areas under the collarbone, about an inch (2.5 cm) out from the middle of the chest. Rub these areas vigorously for 30 seconds to one minute, as you look from left to right.

## BELLY BREATHING
This improves the supply of oxygen to the entire body and relaxes the central nervous system while increasing your energy levels. It can help improve both reading and speaking abilities.

**1.** Put your hands on your abdomen. Exhale through your mouth in short little puffs, as if you are keeping a feather in the air, until your lungs feel empty.

**2.** Inhale deeply through your nose, filling yourself like a balloon beneath your hand. (By arching your back slightly you can take in even more air.)

**3.** Slowly and fully exhale through your mouth.

**4.** Repeat this inhalation and exhalation in a natural rhythm during the course of three or more breaths.

# Part three: spirit

*Where is the spiritual in everyday life? Few of us make time during the working week for spiritual practices: many of us don't even consider our souls during the nine-to-five routine. By the time the evening arrives most of us are too dog-tired to even think about meditation or fostering spiritual awareness: we just want to slump in front of the television.*

*A weekend, though, offers endless spiritual possibilities. In this part we'll explore various approaches to the spirit, none of which asks for any particular faith or religious belief. One weekend is designed to foster spiritual awareness, introducing many key concepts for spiritual work. If you've always wondered about the chakras or wanted to learn how to heal or to read your aura, this is the weekend for you! I firmly believe everyone needs retreats, holidays for the soul, and our Retreat weekend offers you a taster of taking spiritual "time-out".*

*Our other two weekends look at two distinct spiritual traditions which lately have gained hugely in popularity. The Shamanic weekend introduces you to the world of the shamans, giving an insight into such key concepts as journeying and spirit animals. The Qabalah weekend plunges you into this ancient mystical tradition and teaches you the rudiments of the Tree of Life, how to build an inner temple, and how to explore the hidden meanings of the Tarot cards.*

*The processes in this part are very deep and will undoubtedly resonate throughout your life. You may well find that many of the techniques and practices you use on a weekend quietly become part of your everyday life – and that it really isn't so difficult to bring soul into the workday grind after all!*

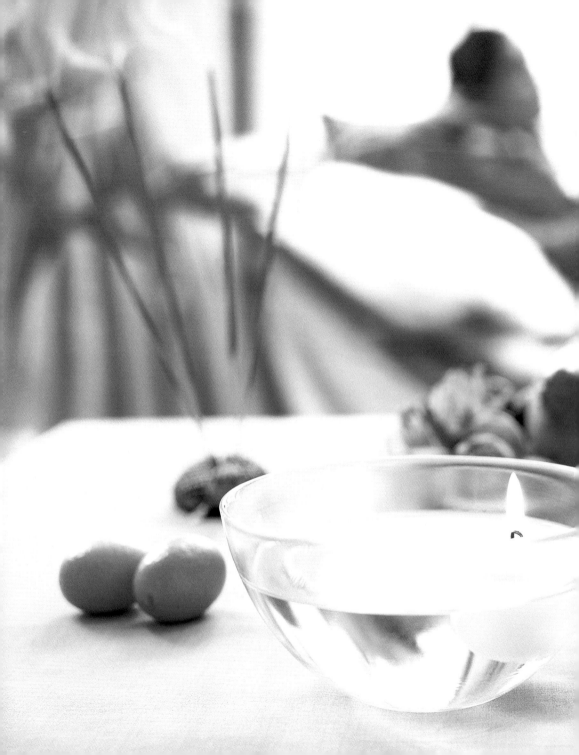

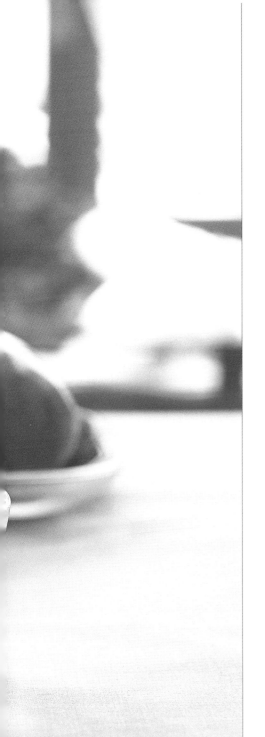

# Retreat weekend

*Sometimes you just need to get away from it all, to go within and re-connect with your essential self. But there's no need to spend loads of money or travel hundreds of miles to a special retreat – just turn your own home into a sanctuary. There is no rigid prescription for a retreat weekend – the following are just some suggestions. Listen to your inner voice and follow your intuition – you won't go wrong.*

*WHAT YOU'LL NEED:*
- *Food – see Food for Retreats (page 93)*
- *Candles, your choice of essential oils, incense*
- *Inspirational books and music (if desired)*
- *Comfortable clothes*
- *Paper, paints, journal, pen*

# Friday evening PREPARE A SANCTUARY

Wind down this evening and make preparations. Arrange
to be by yourself or ask your family for uninterrupted
peace and seclusion. Warn friends you won't be available
for calls or visits. Put a "do not disturb" message on your
answer machine – and your door! Assemble everything
you need so you don't have to go out.

## MAKE YOUR SPACE YOUR OWN
You may want to do the following:
✦ Clear your space of clutter (see page 76 for tips).
✦ Clean it with natural cleansers. Add a few drops of
selected essential oils to make your room smell delicious
and to affect your mood.
✦ Remove everything distracting (television, radio,
computer, any work files, etc.).
✦ Make your space comfortable and relaxing: cushions
and a rug for floorwork; a yoga mat or meditation stool;
a comfortable chair.
✦ Think whether you will want silence or some well-
chosen music (keep tapes or CDs on hand).
✦ Pick out a few inspirational books.
✦ Arrange candles for soft light and to introduce the
element of fire. Pick your favourite aromatherapy oils to
burn or choose incense you like. Surround yourself by
images and objects which inspire you.

## SUPPER
Eat a light, nourishing, soothing supper (see opposite for
ideas). Make your mealtimes mindful: say a form of grace
in thanks for your food. Be aware of each mouthful of
food. Try to eat in silence, concentrating on your food –
don't distract yourself with a book or music.

## CHOOSE YOUR PURPOSE

After supper, sit down in your sanctuary and mull over what you want from this weekend. Affirm to yourself that this is a time for YOU – that it is a sacred time, devoted to your inner wellbeing. You may wish to light a candle and quietly focus on your intention.
Ask yourself:

✦ What do I most need in my life right now?

✦ What does retreating mean to me?

✦ What do I fear about going on retreat?

✦ What do I most hope for on this retreat?

✦ What questions should I ask myself on this retreat?

### FOOD FOR RETREATS

*You need comforting, nourishing food that's balanced (not too soporific but not too stimulating). The best way to do this is to follow macrobiotic guidelines. Choose your foods from this list: • whole grains • beans and legumes • vegetables and fruits, including seaweeds such as dulse, wakame, etc. • seeds and nuts • tofu, tempeh, and miso. Make your choices simple (you don't want to spend ages preparing and cooking): • soups • rice and steamed vegetables • salads with added nuts and seeds if it's warm • vegetable stews and casseroles if it's cold • fruit salads and fruit and vegetable juices.*

# Saturday FOLLOW YOUR SPIRIT

Abandon fixed routine and do as your spirit guides you.
Here are a few guidelines you may find helpful:

✦ Eat three healthy meals a day. You don't have to fast
on a modern retreat – if you're hungry it's tough to
concentrate on anything other than food.

✦ Early to bed, early to rise is a good maxim to follow.

✦ Meditate or quietly contemplate during your day.

✦ Try breathing, yoga, chi kung or tai chi (dip into other
weekends for exercises and routines).

✦ To explore inner issues try painting (see below),
writing, chanting, or dance.

✦ Note down thoughts, images, dreams in your journal.

✦ Try to spend some time in nature – quietly walking,
meditating, doing yoga, or just sitting and observing.

✦ Don't let yourself get too busy!

## PAINTING YOUR INNER SELF

Painting, drawing, and sculpting are all ideal partners in
the retreat process. Don't come with any expectations.
Let go of the concept that you have to paint "properly"
or draw well. Art can free the unconscious mind quite
dramatically, revealing startling answers to problems.

You'll need somewhere you can be messy. Cover an
entire wall with an old sheet and put another on the
floor. Or work on a table or pin your paper to a piece of
chipboard on the wall. Choose large sheets of paper –
newspaper is fine. And pick your choice of art material –
poster paints are a good choice for beginners.

**1.** Spend a moment centring yourself and breathing
deeply. Try full abdominal breathing (page 19).

**2.** Now look at the paper and paints and brushes. Which
brush draws you? Which colour calls to you? Pick up
your brush and make marks on the paper.

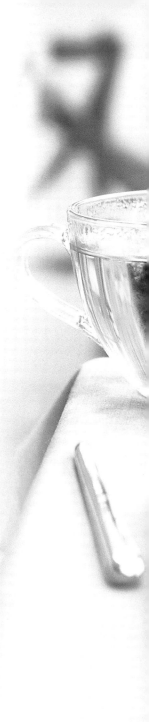

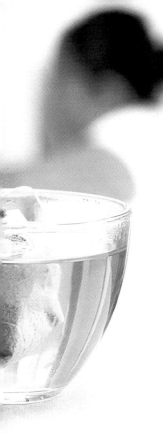

**3.** If an image comes to mind represent it however you like. Or you just splash colour around. Don't worry if it doesn't seem to "go right" – whatever you have done is just fine.

**4.** If you're really stuck try one of these tips: paint with your non-dominant hand; close your eyes and paint; put on some music and follow the rhythm of the sounds.

**5.** Allow your feelings free rein. You may want to use your hands and fingers instead of a brush; or scratch or tear the paper; or simply paint one colour or one tiny image.

**6.** If you feel emotions coming up, allow them space. You may feel like crying, or shouting, or beating the wall (or a cushion).

**7.** When you feel you've finished, take a break. Drink a cup of herbal tea, or eat a meal, or take a quiet walk outside.

**8.** Come back and look at your image. What does it say to you? You could write any thoughts and responses in your journal. If your painting had a name, what would it be? If it had a message for you, what would it be?

---

### MAKING A MANDALA OF YOUR LIFE

✦ *Draw or paint a large circle and put a photo of yourself in the middle.*
✦ *Divide the circle into segments, one for each role in your life, e.g. "lover", "cook", "mother", "partner", "exerciser", "gardener", "software developer", etc. How much time do you give each role? Make it clear by how large each segment is.*
✦ *Now put an image for each role. You may want to cut out images from magazines – or paint pictures, symbols, or just colours.*
✦ *Look at your mandala – how does it make you feel?*
✦ *Now paint a mandala of the way you would LIKE your life to be. How large are the segments now? What other roles would you explore?*

# Sunday SEEKING THE SACRED

Traditionally, retreats are religious in purpose. However you feel about mainstream religion, it is worth bringing a sense of the sacred to your retreat. How you do this is up to you but you might consider building an altar.

## BUILDING AN ALTAR
An altar is simply a place to focus your intentions and open yourself to the possibility of the divine. It can take many forms and should incorporate items which have meaning for you. For example:

✦ Items which symbolize the elements: a bowl of water (you can add flowers or petals); a candle (for fire); incense or aromatherapy burner (for air); crystals or a bowl of salt or pebbles (for earth).

✦ Images, statues, pictures which have meaning for you – these could be religious (a figure of Buddha, the Cross, a Star of David, the Goddess, Shiva, etc.) or secular.

✦ Items from the natural world which resonate – stones from a stream; a pebble or shell; leaves and flowers; pieces of wood.

✦ Pictures of people dear to you; or images of yourself doing activities you enjoy. Or something which symbolizes your goals and aspirations.

## THE WAY OF PRAYER

You can use your altar as a place of prayer – or find another spot which suits you. There are many ways to pray – you may feel comfortable with traditional prayers, chants, or blessings particular to your (present or childhood) faith. But equally you can take a more freeform approach.

✦ If there were a deity, what would you want to ask him/her?

✦ What is there in your life for which you are thankful? What gifts have you been given? Offer up your gratitude for life's blessings.

✦ What is there in life which troubles you? Ask for guidance, help, support, and comfort.

✦ You don't need to sit still, or kneel to pray. Try going on a "prayer walk". Pick somewhere safe and preferably beautiful, where you can walk slowly. Keep your pace measured and rhythmic. Notice the world around you – pay attention to the beauty in nature. As you walk, you may want to pray for people you know; or mull over concerns or anxieties with the divine.

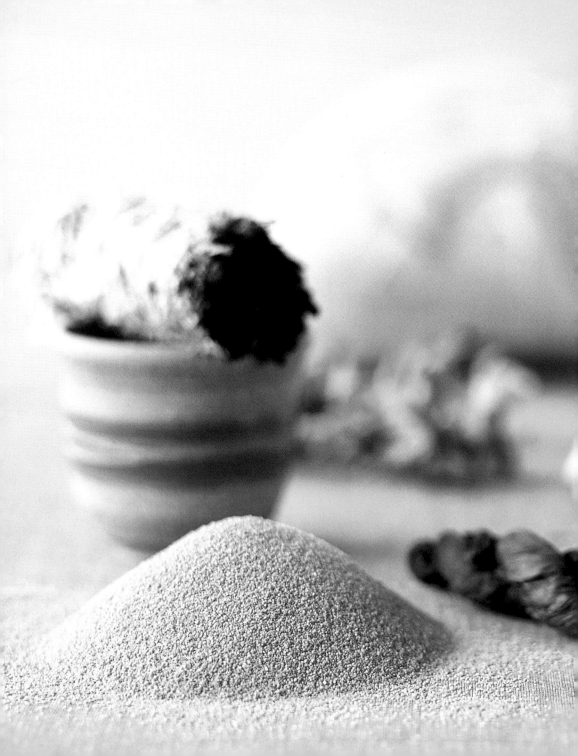

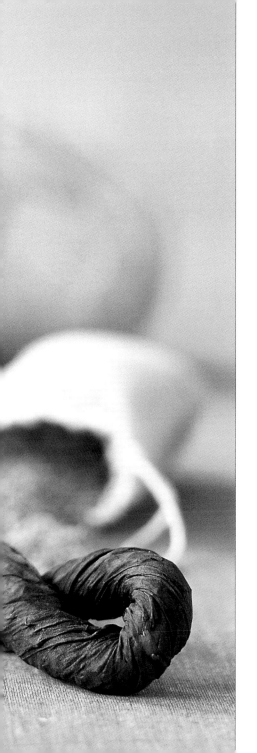

# Shamanic weekend

*Shamans are sacred wisdomkeepers; men and women who can walk between the worlds, talk to animals, and perform deep healing for body and soul. Every ancient culture had shamans – the wise ones still do. We aren't all drawn to the shamanic path in this life (and it is a tough and arduous training) but we can use its teachings to deepen our link with the world around us. This weekend let us walk with the shamans – just for a while.*

*WHAT YOU'LL NEED:*
- *Smudge stick*
- *Feather, shell, sand, or earth*
- *Tape of drumming*
- *Tobacco or cornmeal*
- *Tape recorder (optional)*

# Friday evening PURIFYING SPIRITS

Start by cleansing yourself in a traditional shamanic way – smudging. Smudge sticks contain herbs with magical and spiritual properties; the most traditional are sagebrush and sweetgrass. The spirits of the herbs can help purify people and places, replacing negative energy with fresh positive vibrations.

**1.** Gather your materials in the middle of the room. If you'd like, make an altar (see page 96). Keep a window open for the negative energy to leave by.

**2.** Light your smudge stick. Wait for it to "catch" – you want it to be smoking steadily rather than flaming.

**3.** Stand (with bare feet) and imagine yourself solidly rooted to the Earth (thank Mother Earth for holding you safely in the world).

**4.** Feel your body straighten, as if being pulled up by a string at the top of the head. Feel your connection with the Heavens above and thank Father Sky for giving you inspiration.

**5.** Now waft the smoke with a feather towards your heart and imagine all the negativity being pulled out by the healing smoke.

**6.** Waft the smoke towards each of your other chakras (see pages 110–111). Can you notice any difference as you smudge each chakra?

**7.** Take the smoke over your head and down your arms. Imagine the smudge is lifting away any negativity. Bring it down your back (as best you can) towards the ground.

**8.** Stand solidly again, with the smudge stick between your hands at heart level. Ask for the negativity to leave and for positive energy to replace it.

**9.** Thank the smudge and put it out by gently pressing it into earth.

**10.** Offer a little tobacco or cornmeal as thanks.

### EATING FOR A SHAMANIC WEEKEND

*While you're doing deep shamanic work you need a light diet. Follow these pointers:*

✦ *Eat only fresh, seasonal, vegan produce.*
✦ *Think about where the food comes from? How is it grown? What is its cycle?*
✦ *Try to connect to the spirit of the plant. What is its energy like? Don't worry if you don't get clear ideas.*
✦ *Give deep thanks to the plant or vegetable before eating it. Eat slowly and with mindfulness. Be aware of each mouthful.*
✦ *Drink plenty of fresh water throughout the weekend.*
✦ *Try to avoid tea and coffee. Drink herbal teas instead and, again, try to contact the energy of the herb.*

# Saturday THE FOUR GUARDIANS

Practice yoga (pages 148–151) to become more flexible
and willing to learn, and go outside to try to get in touch
with the energy of a stone or piece of wood (see page 85).
Now meet the four mighty Spirit Animals, or guardians,
of Native American tradition. Find a quiet spot
(preferably outside) and lay out four stones in a large
diamond. Light a smudge stick, smudge yourself, and sit
in the diamond. One by one, call upon the guardians.

**1.** The stone in front of you represents Eagle, guardian of
the East. Far-sighted and protective, he can bring
inspiration, clear thoughts, and decision making.

**2.** The stone behind you represents Bear, guardian of the
West. Powerful and good to have watching your back,
she brings courage and determination and is a strong,
cleansing energy. Bear also governs dreaming.

**3.** To your right sits Coyote, guardian of the South. He's
clever, quick witted (good to have in meetings or when
you need your wits about you), and governs emotions.

**4.** To your left stands Buffalo, guardian of the North.
Dependable and a wonderful grounding energy, she gives
knowledge of Life and Death and bestows wisdom.

**5.** Offer smudge to each guardian, asking for insight and
wisdom. Which guardian's qualities do you need?

**6.** Are you drawn to one guardian? If so, ask permission
to talk to that animal and for guidance. Be respectful.

**7.** Ask if it's time to meet your ally, a personal animal
guide you have a strong bond with. If they feel it's right,
it may "appear" – either literally or in your imagination.
If so, ask its permission to talk to it. Is it "your" animal
(or, rather, are you "its" human!)? Ask if it will become
your guide and protector in life and dreaming.

**8.** Thank the animal and guardians and offer smudge in
thanks. You may also offer tobacco or cornmeal.

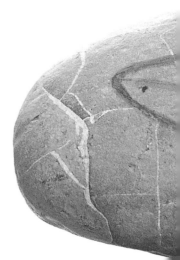

## MEDICINE WALK

*This afternoon, go on a medicine walk and let nature give you valuable teachings.*

✦ *Shower with a few drops of cedarwood oil. Smudge yourself. Don't eat anything.*

✦ *Make a line of stones (or salt) outside your front door and step over it – from now on, everything you see, hear, or touch will be significant until you return and step over the line again.*

✦ *Walk mindfully: feel your feet on the ground and notice the world around – does anything beg for attention (a bird, a flower, a person, an advertisement). Note down everything and ponder the meanings later.*

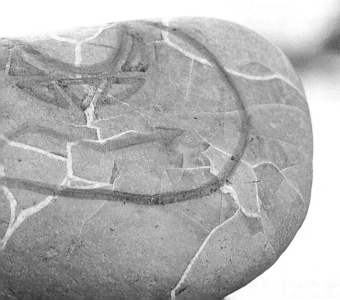

# Sunday SHAMANIC JOURNEY

Don't eat before your journey. Find a warm, comfortable, safe room where you won't be disturbed. If you tape the instructions, leave plenty of pauses.

**1.** Smudge yourself and each corner of the room. Ensure your stick is safe (and won't send out sparks) while you are journeying.

**2.** Lie down and check your body is relaxed from feet to face, tensing and releasing each part.

**3.** Turn on your drumming tape and listen. Where can you feel it in your body? Let your mind follow the beats.

**4.** You're in a beautiful forest. The sun glints through the trees. You can smell the scent of the leaves, the sap, the moist humus under foot.

**5.** Beside you is either your spirit animal or a guardian.

**6.** As you walk, the path widens until you find yourself in a clearing. Ahead is an old, enormous tree.

**7.** You look at it, noticing everything about it. A door is carved into the living tree. As you and your animal approach, it opens in front of you.

**8.** Steps go into the tree – they may go up or down, or further into the tree. Choose whichever path seems right (you can ask your animal for advice) and go to the end.

**9.** You enter one of the three shamanic realms (see box). Watch everything you see – people, animals, birds, plants, or trees. Approach with great respect and ask for any message they have for you. You might even find parts of yourself! Thank any creature that helps you.

**10.** When you feel ready, go back to the steps and return to the ground. Walk back through the forest, feeling yourself returning to waking awareness.

**11.** Gently open your eyes. Sit quietly for a few minutes. When you're ready, get up and stamp your feet. Now drink and eat something. Record your experiences.

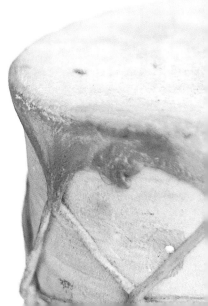

**THE THREE REALMS**

THE LOWER WORLD: *the Place of Death but not a dark, frightening place. You may meet animals here or souls of your ancestors, or parts of your soul which have become lost or cut off. You might invite these parts to rejoin you.*

THE MIDDLE WORLD: *a parallel world to this one where you'll find information and answers about this world and life, and where you can see people, animals, and places that exist now. You can ask for information to help you understand people and situations better.*

THE UPPER WORLD: *a world of clouds and light, filled with angels and spirits. You can gain knowledge from these higher beings. You can ask for spiritual wisdom and advice – if they are willing to talk to you.*

**GET STEAMED!**

*After all the inner work you've been doing try to have a steam at a gym or Turkish bath. (Only go to a sweat lodge run by a highly experienced shaman.) As you steam, envisage negativity leaving you. Afterwards, in your heightened state of awareness, you may meet a guide or make a journey with your animal.*

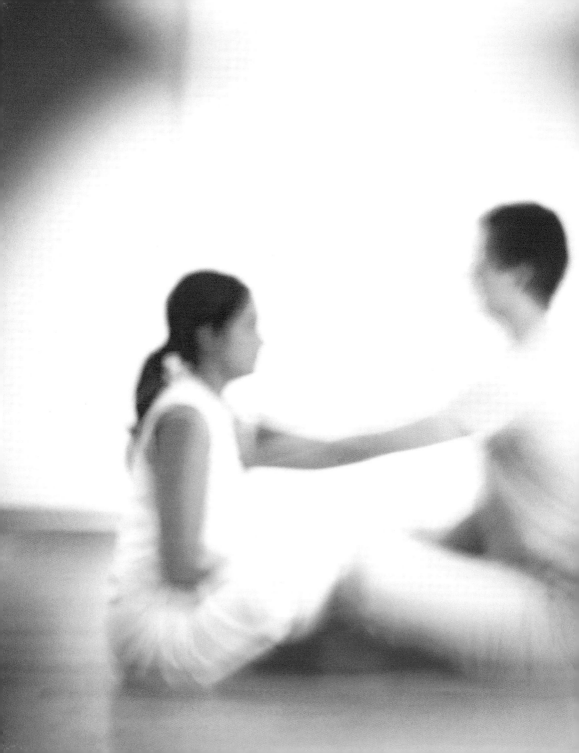

# Spiritual awareness

*Should you feel the need for a more spiritual way of life, this weekend could be the answer. It introduces many key concepts of spiritual development and teaches you how to put them into practice. You will discover more about how to sense vital energy in the body, and how to work with your chakras and auras. The result should be a far better balance in your life between body, mind, and spirit.*

**WHAT YOU'LL NEED:**
- *Essential oils: rosemary, eucalyptus, and lavender*
- *Sea salt*
- *Paper (or journal) and pen*

# Friday evening SENSING VITAL ENERGY

Let's start by learning how to sense vital energy in the body. This is the key to much of the work we will do over the weekend.

**1.** Take off your shoes and stand with your feet shoulder-width apart. Feel your knees soft and your shoulders relaxed. You feel as if your head were being gently pulled up towards the ceiling, lengthening out your neck.

**2.** Now close your eyes and just become aware of your breath. Stand and breathe for a few minutes, becoming aware that, as you relax, you're breathing more deeply and slowly. Focus your attention on your solar plexus, just above your navel. Try to breathe into this area, the centre of your Self.

**3.** You will soon start to feel a tingling of energy around the body. The more you relax and breathe, the more noticeable it will become. We will build on this through the weekend.

## MEANING OF SPIRITUALITY

Spend time this evening thinking about what spirituality means to you. You might ask yourself:

✦ Do you have a particular religion or faith?

✦ Was your family religious or non-religious?

✦ How do you react to the idea of spirituality? What words come to mind?

✦ Where can we find spirit and soul?

✦ Do you think we possess the ability to heal?

✦ What do you believe happens to us after death?

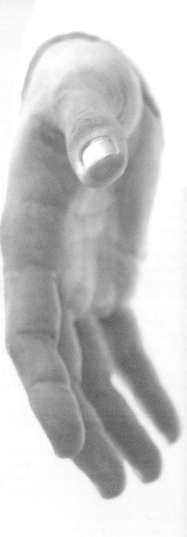

## HEALING HANDS

Try activating the healing power in your hands.

**1.** Rub your palms together vigorously for a minute.

**2.** Hold your palms a few inches apart, as if you were holding a small ball. Is there a tingling or warmth coming from your hands? Now "bounce" your hands and feel the energy pulse as you move your hands in and out.

**3.** Hold your hands slightly further apart, as if you were holding a larger ball. Imagine that in the middle of one palm is a circular area that can send healing energy. Rub this spot with the thumb of your other hand: you are opening up this area.

**4.** Repeat on the other hand.

**5.** If you want to send healing energy you can hold your hand or hands over a part of the body, or a chakra (see next page) and visualize healing energy pouring into your body from the top of your head and streaming out through the healing spots on your hands.

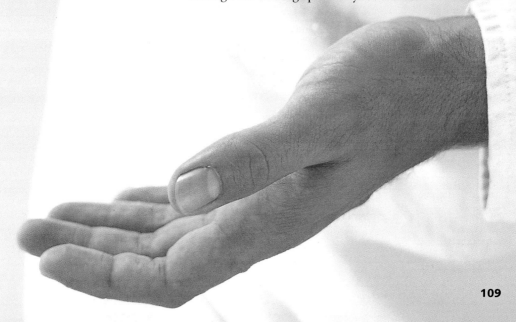

# Saturday EXPERIENCING CHAKRAS

Start the day with the spiritual Sun Salutation (pages
148–149) and then investigate your chakras.

### ENERGY CENTRES

According to Vedic philosophy we possess seven major
energy centres, or chakras, from above our heads to the
base of the spine. This exercise helps you become aware
of their energy moving within you. If chakras are new to
you do the exercise and write down your experiences or
feelings and then read the box opposite to find out more.
If you find visualization easy use a different colour for
each chakra. Otherwise, stick to white for each.

**1.** Take off your shoes and stand as you did in Friday's
opening exercise. Relax your body, close your eyes, and
focus on your breathing.

**2.** Imagine a shining white sphere of pure energy above
your head. This crown chakra is violet. Breathe into that
ball of light for a few breaths: how does it feel?

**3.** On your last breath, as you breathe out, bring your
attention to the sphere (indigo) in the forehead. Breathe
into this sphere and notice how its energy feels.

**4.** Once again, as you breathe out, descend to the throat
chakra (blue). Notice the different energy here and
breathe it in before continuing.

**5.** Move to the heart chakra (green). Spend some time at
this important centre.

**6.** Move to the solar plexus chakra (yellow).

**7.** Between the lower abdomen and the navel is the sacral
chakra (orange).

**8.** Bring your breath down to the base chakra (deep red),
at the base of the spine. Breathe here for a few minutes.

**9.** Finally, imagine a lightning flash descends from above,
through all the chakras, energizing your entire body.

**THE CHAKRAS**
*CROWN: concerns understanding, connection with the Divine. Strengthen with meditation, prayer, visiting sacred places.*
*BROW: concerns imagination, intuition, dreams, insights. Strengthen with art therapy, dreamwork, meditation.*
*THROAT: concerns communication, creativity. Strengthen with voicework, singing, shouting, bodywork or massage, honest communication.*
*HEART: concerns love, intimacy, balance, relationships. Strengthen with pranayama (yogic breathing), journaling, psychotherapy to relieve old hurts, acceptance of yourself.*
*SOLAR PLEXUS: concerns self-esteem, inner strength, confidence, will power. Strengthen with stress management, deep relaxation, martial arts, Pilates.*
*SACRAL: concerns sexuality, sensuality, partnerships. Strengthen with listening to music, dance, bodywork, emotional work.*
*BASE: concerns the material world, physical body, social standing. Strengthen with exercise, massage, yoga, gardening, pottery.*

**EVENING RITUAL**
*Do the Moon Salutation (pages 150–151). End the day with a bath, a symbol of rebirth and cleansing to body and soul.*
*✦ Add two tablespoons of salt to the running water.*
*✦ When the bath is full, add one drop each of rosemary, eucalyptus, and lavender.*
*✦ Lie back and feel cleansed of negativity.*

# Sunday SEEING AURAS

Start once again with the Sun Salutation (see pages 148–149) and a period of quiet meditation or prayer before investigating auras.

**WHAT THE AURA COLOURS MEAN**
*These are the most common meanings:*
**PURPLE:** *mysticism, spirituality*
**INDIGO:** *wisdom, sensitivity*
**BLUE:** *intelligence, control, intuition*
**GREEN:** *kindness, caring, gentleness, balance*
**YELLOW:** *fun, optimism, joy, vitality*
**ORANGE:** *warmth, generosity, vitality*
**RED:** *ambition, sexuality, vitality*
**PINK:** *shyness, modesty, gentleness, love*
**BLACK:** *depression, anxiety, fear, illness*
**GREY:** *depression, fear, low energy*
**BROWN:** *negativity, materialistic*
**WHITE:** *illness, exhaustion or (from crown) spiritual awareness*

## SHIMMERING ENERGY

The aura is the area of vital energy that vibrates around our bodies. It can show a great deal about our physical, mental, and spiritual health. Learning how to see auras is actually very simple.
**1.** Start by looking at a tree or healthy plant. Slightly unfocus your eyes and you should start to see a shimmering around the tree or plant.

**2.** Now try seeing the aura of an animal. You can even give your pets "aura strokes" by stroking about an inch (2.5 cm) above their fur (cats, in particular, love this).
**3.** If you want to see someone else's aura, stand about 10 feet (3 m) away and look past their shoulders and head, again unfocusing the eyes. You should see a fuzzy light. If you look past this you may start to see colours – this takes some practice.

### SENSING A SACRED SPACE

Visit a sacred space – either a building or somewhere in nature. Spend time just being there. Notice what you feel and what you sense. Try feeling the energy with your energized hands. Can you notice any particular chakra being activated? If you are outside, do you see the aura surrounding the trees, or water, or stones?

When you return home do something physical: cleaning is ideal. It is very easy to become seduced into thinking that the spiritual is all airy-fairy, beautiful, and lofty: but in truth you can find true spirit in the lowliest places, too. Try to turn your cleaning into spiritual practice: invest it with care and meaning.

### EVENING FOCUS

Do the Moon Salutation (see pages 150–151) again and spend some time focusing on breathing (check out the exercises on pages 19, 26, 40, and 87).

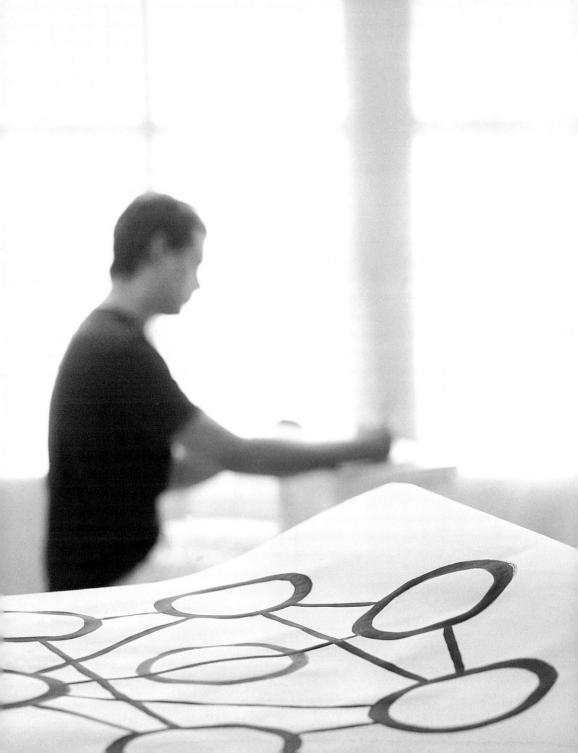

# Qabalah weekend

*The Qabalah is Jewish in origin but has been embraced by mystics from all races and religions. It offers a map to Creation, from the first intention of God to the physical reality of life on Earth. A true study of the Qabalah is a lifetime's work but this weekend should give you a taste of its teachings and their applications.*

*WHAT YOU'LL NEED:*
- *Paper and pens*
- *A compass or small jar to draw around*
- *Pack of Tarot cards (the Rider Waite pack is ideal for beginners, but choose some with illustrations that appeal to you).*

# Friday evening THE TREE OF LIFE

Get to know the Tree of Life, the central map of the Qabalah. The best way is to draw it by copying the illustration on this page on to a large piece of paper. Draw the Tree several times until you become familiar with the names of the eleven sephirah and their positions.

**1** MALKUTH The Kingdom. Governs: the body, the Earth, and the material, physical world. Colours: yellow, olive, russet and black flecked with gold. Symbols: the equal-armed cross, a double cube, and the magic circle.

**2** YESOD The Foundation. Governs: the subconscious, our past, our future potential, our sexual nature, the Moon. Colours: indigo, violet, and very dark purple. Symbols: perfumes and sandals.

**3** HOD Glory. Governs: the mind, intellect, willpower, communication, magic, and spells. Colours: violet, purple, and orange. Symbol: the apron.

**4** NETZACH Victory. Governs: feelings, creative art, nature. Colours: amber, emerald, and olive flecked with gold. Symbols: the rose, the lamp, and the girdle.

**5** TIPHARETH Beauty. Governs: the Self, the ego, the soul – pure self-awareness. Often known as the "Christ Centre" for its lesson of true love and sacrifice. Colours: rose-pink, yellow, and rich, salmon pink. Symbols: the cross, the cube, and a truncated pyramid.

**6** GEBURAH Severity. Governs: judgement, unmitigated truth, personal will and power, strength, order, activity, and focused awareness. Colours: orange, bright red, and scarlet. Symbols include the pentagon, the sword, the spear, and the scourge.

**7** CHESED Mercy (sometimes known as Love). Governs: balanced feelings of caring, sensitivity, and co-operation. Colours: deep violets, purples, and blue. Symbols: the orb, the wand, and the sceptre.

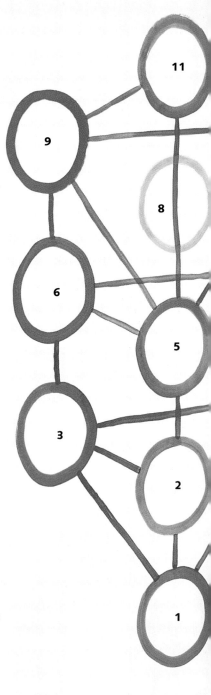

**116**

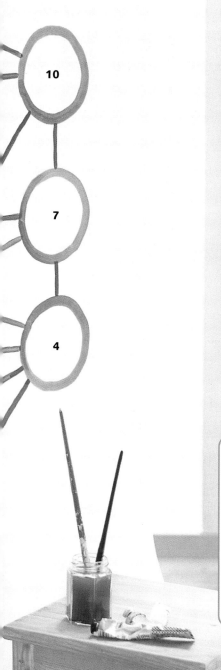

**8** DAATH Knowledge. The one sephirah not situated on the Tree; it is the mysterious hidden sephiroth that lies in the middle of the Abyss, above Tiphareth and below Kether. Governs: all the unresolved and irrational elements of the psyche. Colours: silver and ultra-violet. Symbols: an empty throne and a silver mirror.

**9** BINAH Understanding. Governs: spiritual awareness and love, the healing power of pure sorrow, and the primal feminine energy. Colours: crimson, black, and dark brown. Symbols: the cup or chalice.

**10** CHOCKMAH Wisdom. Governs: spiritual will and purpose and the primal masculine force. Colours: soft blues and greys. Symbols: all phallic symbols – standing stones, the tower, and the rod of power.

**11** KETHER The Crown. The fount of Creation, where life begins, where there is no distinction between male and female or between energy and matter. Colours: pure white brilliance and white flecked with gold. Symbol: the equal-armed cross.

---

### AN EVENING PRAYER
*Before you go to bed, say the Qabalistic cross, a non-denominational form of blessing and protection.*
**1.** *Stand facing East with your feet firmly on the floor*
**2.** *Touch your forehead and say, "To Thee, Oh God"*
**3.** *Touch your solar plexus and say, "Be the Kingdom"*
**4.** *Touch your right shoulder and say, "And the Power"*
**5.** *Touch your left shoulder and say, "And the Glory"*
**6.** *Clasp your hands together over your chest and say, "For ever and ever. Amen"*

# Saturday AWAKEN THE MIDDLE PILLAR

This morning you are going to activate the Tree of Life within you by awakening the Middle Pillar sephirah.

**1.** Stand facing towards the East.

**2.** Visualize a shining sphere of bright white light (Kether) floating above your head.

**3.** As a beam of white lights shoots from this sphere down into your head intone the word EHEIEH (Eh-hay-yay) slowly several times. Imagine the name vibrating over and through your head.

**4.** As the beam descends into your throat it spreads out to become a glowing sphere of gleaming white. Intone the name JEHOVAH ELOHIM (Ye-ho-vah El-oh-heem). Let the name vibrate through your neck and throat.

**5.** The light shoots down to your solar plexus and again settles into a glowing white sphere. Intone the name JEHOVAH ALOAH VA DAATH (Ye-ho-vah El-oh-vay Da-art) – feel the energy warm and activate this area.

**6.** As the light descends to your genitals intone the name SHADDAI EL CHAI (Shad-ee El Key). The "key" syllable is guttural, like the "ch" in loch. Feel the energy pulsing here.

**7.** Finally the light pours down your legs to your feet, forming a large sphere reaching into the Earth below. Imagine this sphere is rooting you to the Earth and intone the name ADONAI HA ARETZ (A-don-ee Ha A-retz).

**8.** Visualize the entire column of light linking you to Heaven above and Earth below. This powerful exercise helps you feel balanced and centred. Repeat it often.

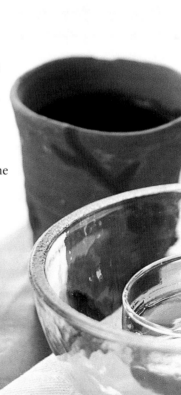

## THE INNER TEMPLE

Each sephiroth has a temple and an attendant archangel. Spend some time building the inner temple of Malkuth. Sit or lie down somewhere undisturbed, comfortable, and shut your eyes. Check your body is relaxed and free from tensions. Focus on your breathing.

**1.** Gradually become aware the floor is cool to your bare feet and made up of black and white tiles laid out in a chequerboard fashion.

**2.** You realize you're in a square-shaped temple which is clear and beautiful. On three walls are large, stained-glass windows: one has a bull, one an eagle, one a lion.

**3.** In the centre stands an altar: two cubes of black wood, one on top of the other, covered with a plain linen cloth. On top sits a bowl of blue crystal within which a light burns, a cup of wine, a loaf of bread, and some ears of corn. Above, a censer burns a fragrant, earthy incense.

**4.** In front of you is a wall with three heavy oak doors without locks or handles. Before the doors are two pillars stretching from floor to ceiling: the one on the left is black ebony; the one on the right is made of pure silver.

**5.** Walk around the temple, looking at the altar, the pillars, the stained-glass windows.

**6.** When you're ready ask to meet the temple's guardian, the archangel Sandalphon. He is tall and his long robe is coloured with gold, earthy brown, soft green, and russet red. His face is gentle and wise, but tinged with sadness.

**7.** Ask him to help you learn wisdom and some of the lessons of Malkuth. Ask him why he is sad (would YOU be sad if you were the archangel of the Earth?).

**8.** When you're ready, say farewell and become aware of waking reality. Open your eyes, stamp your feet, and have something to eat.

**119**

# Sunday

Take the morning off and go outside for a walk in nature.
Become aware of the earth energy of Malkuth around
you. Do you notice the energy of any other sephiroth?
Maybe you recall a dream (Yesod) or find yourself filled
with love for your child (Tiphareth); or feel censorious
about something you read in the newspaper (Geburah).
Start applying the Tree to every part of your life.

## TAROT PLAY

Become accustomed to your Tarot cards. Separate out the
Major Arcana – which images are particularly appealing
or disturbing? Pick the card which jumps out at you most
of all and sit quietly and meditate on its picture. What
does it say to you? What are its associations? Do you like
the card, or not? Why? You may want to write down
your thoughts – or paint images or colours.

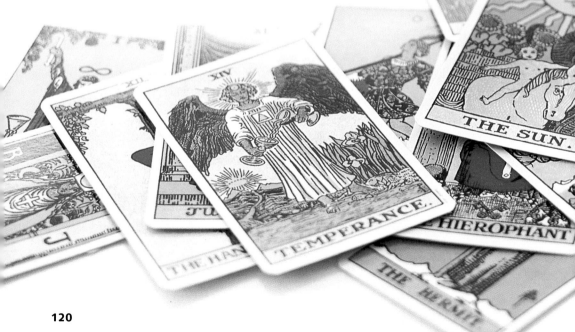

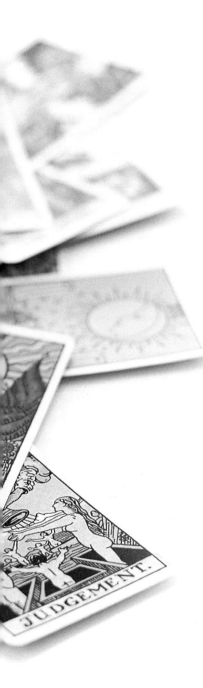

## PATHWORKING

Go on a journey through your chosen Tarot card. All the Major Arcana cards are represented on the Tree of Life so you will be doing what is known as a "pathworking", travelling from one sephiroth to another. You can start your journey from the temple of Malkuth.

**1.** Build up the temple as you did yesterday and ask Sandalphon for help to travel to your path.

**2.** The image of your chosen card is embroidered on an enormous curtain that stretches across the two pillars. Look at every detail. As you walk closer you notice the image is alive and moving. The edges seem to blur.

**3.** Sandalphon invites you forwards and you step into and through the curtain. You might notice a rushing, as if you were being sucked upwards in an elevator (you may even pass through some of the sephirah) – then you step out into the landscape of your card.

**4.** What happens next? Whom do you meet? Do you feel compelled to walk through the landscape? What do you learn?

**5.** When you feel ready to return, turn around and see the card once again hanging like a curtain. Walk towards it and through it once more, back into the Earth Temple.

**6.** Spend some time discussing your journey with Sandalphon, who may give some illumination.

**7.** Thank him and notice your body on the floor and slowly return to waking reality. Stamp your feet and have a warm drink and something to eat to ground you fully.

# Part four: seasonal

*In the past our ancestors followed the yearly cycle of the seasons with inordinate care and attention. The earth and its rhythms are essential when you rely on its bounty for your everyday survival and so – even until quite recently – people honoured the shifting energy of the year with a round of festivals and rituals.*

*Nowadays, few of us rely on the earth directly for our daily bread and meat – we are simply not part of the farming process when we buy our food from a supermarket! We even lock ourselves away from the elements in our centrally heated, air-conditioned homes and offices, rarely venturing out into the world of nature. This disassociation from the earth's cycle is a great loss for modern humans. Nature moves from the quiet of Winter to new life in Spring; from the full abundance of Summer to the slow decline of Autumn. Whether we like it or not, our own lives, too, follow this annual cycle and so the celebrations and rituals of the passing year can help to bring us into harmony with our spiritual and emotional needs.*

*The four weekends in this part help to ease us into the distinctive energy of each of the major seasons. They are a means of signifying to the psyche that it is time for a shift, a change. In each weekend you will learn how and what to eat seasonally, and how to build an altar to celebrate and welcome the new seasonal energy.*

*You will also discover what kind of issues need to be dealt with at these changing times of the year – and will be shown easy processes with which to work. There are also plenty of fun suggestions for how to enjoy each and every season.*

# Welcoming Spring

*The days are getting longer, the evenings lighter, nature is in a flurry of activity and new growth: everything is ALIVE and ready to burst through. So your weekend should be a celebration of fresh new life, joy, and energy. Start by clearing your space and spring cleaning it with fresh citrus oils. And you can gently shed some of the extra layers you've accumulated over the Winter.*

*WHAT YOU'LL NEED:*
- *Food for Spring (see page 127)*
- *Essential oils: lemon, orange, bergamot, or tangerine*
- *Spring flowers, incense (optional)*
- *Pale green cloth, green candles*
- *Eggs and dyes or paints*
- *Your choice of items for your altar*
- *Magazines, scissors, recent photo of yourself, glue, and a large sheet of paper*

# Saturday THE JOYS OF SPRING

Get up early, stretch, and perform the Sun Salutation (see pages 148–149). Go for a walk while the dew is still on the ground and collect some of nature's Spring bounty: flowers, catkins, branches with buds, a special stone that cries for your attention. Notice the fresh air and sense the clean, invigorating energy of Spring.

### SPRING ALTAR
Come back, shower (with two drops of essential oil), and eat a light breakfast. Then make your Spring altar.
**1.** Use a pale green altar cloth to reflect the shades of fresh new buds. Choose green candles, too.
**2.** Evaporate fresh citrus scents in your aromatherapy burner – or burn a light, fresh incense.
**3.** Arrange the items you collected outside and place a vase of Spring flowers beside them.

**4.** Spring is a time of rising fertility and sexual energy so celebrate this energy at your altar with old fertility symbols such as painted eggs. You can paint your wishes for the year on to the eggs. Or experiment with natural dyes: an onion in the boiling water will turn the eggs a delicate yellow.
**5.** Add some seeds you will soon be planting now the earth is warming up (either literal plant seeds or pieces of paper with your desires for the year written on them).

## SEASONAL WINDOW BOX

Think about where you want your box and choose your plants accordingly. A box outside your kitchen could provide handy culinary herbs, such as basil, chives, parsley, sage or rosemary (you will eventually need to transfer the last two as they will grow big).

If you have a small yard or balcony consider starting your own vegetable patch – or planting a few vegetables in a gro-bag.

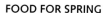

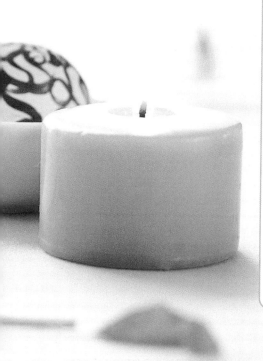

### FOOD FOR SPRING

*Now is the time to shed any extra weight you put on over the Winter. But do it gently and not by jumping into a draconian diet – Spring can suffer winds that are cold and unpredictable so you still need to nourish your body.*

✦ *Make the most of the fresh Spring greens and vegetables to make lighter but still warming fare: stir-fries, soups, warm salads, frittata (vegetable omelettes).*

✦ *Fish, chicken, and turkey are good protein sources and work well with Spring vegetables.*

✦ *Avoid sweets and sugary snacks – they will stress your body.*

✦ *If you can, shift from drinking coffee and tea and try herbal teas instead.*

✦ *If you're feeling run down, take a daily, good-quality multi-vitamin and mineral supplement. You might also visit a medical herbalist for an individualized tonic.*

# Sunday EXPRESSING YOURSELF

Once again, perform the Sun Salutation (see pages 148–149) and take a walk before breakfast. This morning, you will really wake up your energy with a home dance class. In the afternoon you're going to explore nature and in the evening you'll be making a Treasure Map.

### EXPRESSIVE DANCING

It doesn't matter whether you're a great dancer or have absolutely no sense of rhythm – you are celebrating Spring in your own way (and nobody need see!). Play a piece of music which symbolizes Spring to you and then dance – if you can dance outside, that's fantastic – but your front room with the curtains drawn will suffice.

Feel your feet solidly on the ground. Rotate your hips to loosen them and to free up your pelvic region. How does your body want to move? Don't be inhibited – just move in whatever way you feel is right. If you find yourself stuck, think about these suggestions:

✦ How would a plant feel coming up into the fresh air after a winter underground?

✦ How are the animals feeling now the days are getting warmer and the living is getter easier?

✦ How would a tree feel when its sap starts to rise?

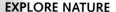

### EXPLORE NATURE

Get outside and enjoy the elements. Go for a long walk in the country or fly a kite on your nearest hilltop! Ride a horse and see the land from a new perspective (wildlife is never as nervous when you're on a horse). Dress up warmly and expect the odd downpour. If it does rain, play with it and see it as a blessing. Fun is an essential part of Spring so indulge yourself – go to the park, visit the zoo, or build a hut in the woods.

### TREASURE MAP

By now you're feeling energized but a bit tired so enjoy a quiet evening making a Treasure Map. Eat a light supper and pour yourself a glass of wine or fruit juice. Light a green candle and burn some oils. Select magazines that you like and tear out images that "speak to your soul" – of your ideal home, of people doing your ideal job, or enjoying themselves in exactly the way you would like. They can either be graphic or evoke a mood or feeling.

Now look through these images more discriminatingly. Which do you REALLY want? Be careful: this powerful exercise has a curious way of coming true.

Arrange your final images on a large piece of paper with a picture of yourself in the middle and whoever you want to share your ideal life beside you. You can include affirmations and words but don't be too prescriptive.

Place your Treasure Map where you will see it every day (opposite your desk or on the kitchen wall is ideal). Your subconscious works in images and so will try to find a way of bringing these images into your life – although expect the unexpected!

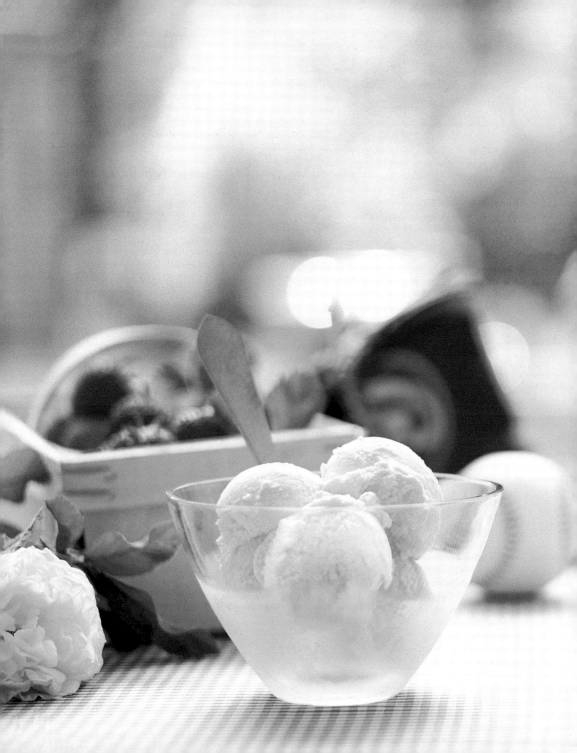

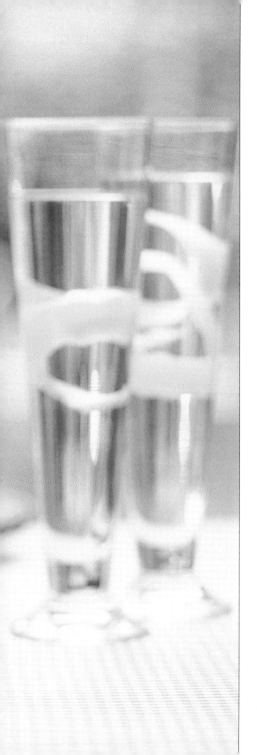

# Welcoming Summer

*Summer is sun-time, fun-time, the exuberant outdoor season of play, holidays, and relaxation – or so it should be! If your Summer is a slog and the living "isn't easy" then take this opportunity to celebrate the joy of the season. Traditionally, the best time would be around the Summer Solstice but any weekend is a good enough excuse.*

*WHAT YOU'LL NEED:*
- *Picnic paraphernalia – your choice of food (see page 132), drink, musical instruments, games, etc.*
- *Bright cloth for your altar, plus colourful candles and your choice of party gear, photographs, etc.*
- *Elm Bach flower remedy*

# Saturday LIGHT, BRIGHT, AND OPENING UP

Make a list of your very favourite people. Call them all up and tell them you love them and want to see them – and how about a big picnic on Sunday?

## SUMMER ALTAR

Spend the morning making your Summer altar – it's a joyous celebration of fun so think wild and unrestrained.
**1.** Choose a bright altar cloth – vivid pink (maybe sari fabric?) or red (the brighter the better) or something crazily patterned or a riot of colour.
**2.** Candles can be any bright colour (but include red).
**3.** Summer fruits and flowers – a profusion of scents and colours. If you can, add the magical midsummer herbs of mugwort, vervain, St John's wort, and thyme.
**4.** Pictures of your favourite people – include those who act as inspiration even though you don't know them.
**5.** Add toys or cartoon figures – maybe party squeakers or balloons – anything that signifies life and joy to you.
**6.** If your altar is not fragrant enough burn some feelgood oils such as geranium or rose.

---

**FOOD FOR SUMMER**
*Adapt your diet to the hotter weather:*
✦ *Lighter, cooler foods.*
✦ *Fresh salads with interesting dressings; fresh fish or chicken barbecued or pan-fried over an open fire, vegetable kebabs and couscous.*
✦ *Summer fruits: eat raw, chop into salads, juice into smoothies with live yogurt.*
✦ *Avoid salty and fatty foods.*
✦ *Drink plenty of water and keep alcohol to a minimum.*

---

## COLD HANDS/FEET
*You're suppressing your feelings, afraid to break the rules, or feel you don't deserve what you want. Think and talk about it.*

## GET IN TOUCH WITH YOUR BODY

Summer is the time to get in touch with both your body and emotions – and to look at how the two are entwined. Any aches, pains, or physical problems you have may be explained physiologically but they may also be an early warning of something going wrong with our psychological wellbeing. It's worth pondering a deeper meaning. Below are suggestions for some common complaints. If yours isn't here, ask yourself what it might mean…your intuition may well have the answer.

## BLUSHING
*You're frightened of what others will think. You're caught between what you want and what you think others require of you. Acknowledge your fear and your desires. Be candid about your concerns and explain why you blush.*

## STIFF NECK
*Someone is treating you unfairly; you feel irritable or upset by someone (or by your own behaviour). Who or what is a "pain in the neck" for you? Write a letter to that person – you don't have to send it. Have a massage or osteopathy for short-term relief.*

## SORE THROAT
*You're not saying what you feel or think. Try to express your feelings. Sing or chant or try screaming or groaning. Consider assertiveness training – or take up a martial art.*

## CYSTITIS
*You feel resentment, anger, disappointment. What or who makes you angry? Express your feelings – if not verbally, then write a letter, paint a picture, or hit a cushion.*

## LOW BACK PAIN
*You're overburdened, overly responsible, or overwhelmed. Put some fun back into your life. Delegate your responsibilities. Take Elm Bach flower remedy.*

# Sunday THE ULTIMATE PICNIC

Give the whole day over to the wild and wonderful picnic (see page 152) you've been planning for all your favourite people. Choose a good spot with water nearby – by the sea, on the shore of a lake, or by a river bank.

Make your preparations. Everyone can join in (it's more fun that way). Choose all the kind of picnic party food you loved as a child (plus a little fragrant punch or the odd bottle of chilled white wine!). So think about small sandwiches, pies, and jellies; or a huge outdoor cookout – maybe a vast paella bubbling over a cookfire or fragrant Moroccan kebabs sizzling on a grill.

Pack plenty of sun cream and big hats. You might have a "theme" for your picnic such as Southern belles and gentlemen or an Edwardian seaside; or Woodstock revisited or Teddy Bears picnic, etc. Children love dressing up and adults often do, too!

You might want to add some props for games – balls, bats, nets (but also allow space for imagination). Also add in musical instruments (if you play them).

**LET THE FUN BEGIN!**

Once you've made your preparations allow your picnic to run itself. Just let people enjoy themselves and relax. Remember it doesn't have to be perfect – the perfection comes from the mix of the right people! Be prepared for some conflicts – Summer is a time of heightened emotion and at pagan ceremonies it's traditional to have mock battles and fights at this time of year.

Maybe work in some physical, competitive games such as tug-of-war or split people into teams and send them on a treasure hunt (perhaps having to find a natural object for every letter of the alphabet). Take it in turns to look after children so you all get a rest.

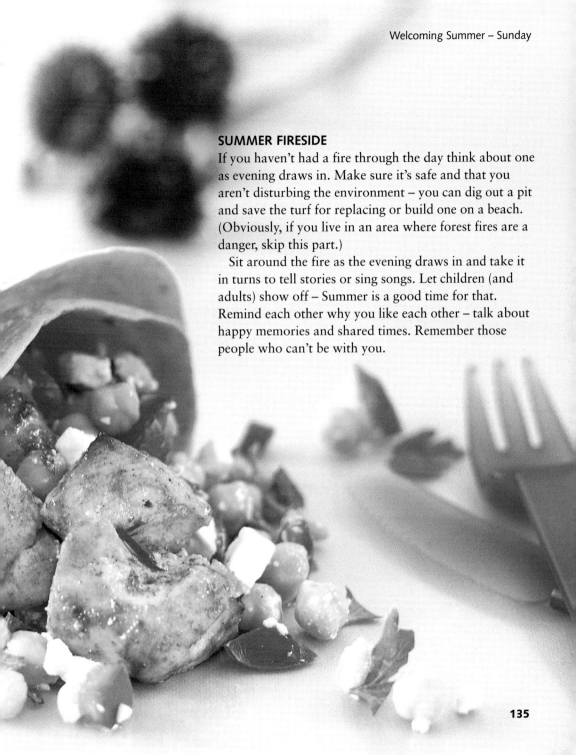

## SUMMER FIRESIDE

If you haven't had a fire through the day think about one as evening draws in. Make sure it's safe and that you aren't disturbing the environment – you can dig out a pit and save the turf for replacing or build one on a beach. (Obviously, if you live in an area where forest fires are a danger, skip this part.)

Sit around the fire as the evening draws in and take it in turns to tell stories or sing songs. Let children (and adults) show off – Summer is a good time for that. Remind each other why you like each other – talk about happy memories and shared times. Remember those people who can't be with you.

**135**

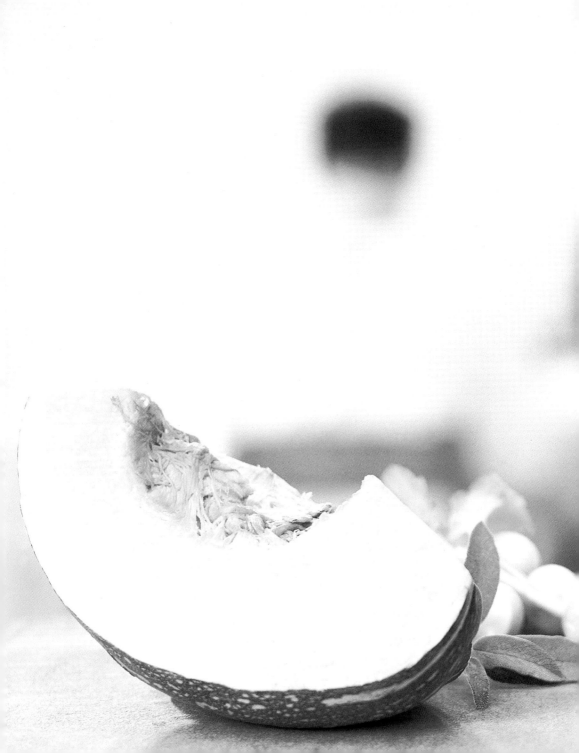

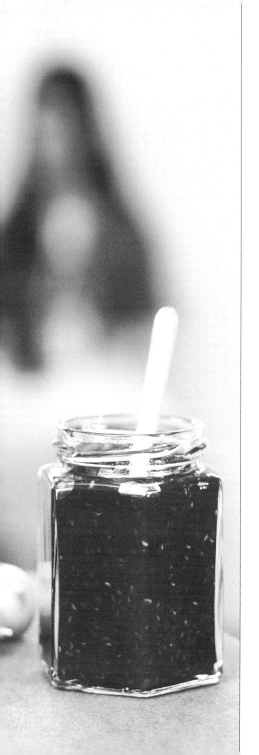

# Welcoming Autumn

*Autumn is a time of contraction, when the earth energy begins to withdraw and pull back below the surface. It's a time for storing what is needed and getting rid of what is no longer necessary for your life. Autumn is a time to regain clarity in your life – for dumping the baggage, both physical and emotional, you have accumulated throughout the year.*

*WHAT YOU'LL NEED:*
- *Food for Autumn (see page 138)*
- *Essential oils: patchouli, pine, cedarwood*
- *Place-cards – or sheets of card*
- *Trash bags or boxes (for unwanted items)*
- *Tape recorder (optional), paper and pen*
- *Candles: yellow and dark green (orange or red are optional)*
- *Yellow tablecloth (optional)*
- *Your choice of items for your altar*

# Saturday ENJOYING THE FRUITS OF THE EARTH

Spend the morning thoroughly clearing and cleaning your home. Open your door and literally (and symbolically) brush the old and unwanted out of your home. Play music to make the task more fun – something rousing and energetic. Clear out your food cupboards, ditching anything that is old or past its sell-by date. Remember herbs and spices lose their potency quite swiftly – throw unwanted herbs on to the last barbecue or the first fire.

Put away your summer clothes and equipment. Make sure it is all clean and in good working order. If it isn't, make a pile of things which need mending and undertake to clear that pile over the next week.

Find recipes for preserving – few of us now prepare our own stores for the harsh months yet making jams, jellies, chutneys, and preserves is a great way of connecting with the energy of Autumn. There's nothing to beat the sight of a larder or cabinet stocked with homemade goodies.

**FOOD FOR AUTUMN**
*Prepare your body for the approach of Winter, with warm, moist, well-lubricated foods that combine sweet and sour tastes.*
*✦ Enjoy fruits (berries, apples, pears, rhubarb, etc.) and start gently stewing or poaching fruit.*
*✦ Vegetables should be steamed or stir-fried. Stuff and bake pumpkins and other squashes.*
*✦ Enjoy warming soups, stews, chowders, broths. Add lentils, other legumes, grains, potatoes.*
*✦ Choose natural sweeteners such as fruit juices, honey, maple syrup, and molasses.*
*✦ Eat fresh nuts (chestnuts, filberts, hazelnuts, walnuts) but sparingly if you're losing weight!*

### AUTUMN ALTAR

Choose a suitable place for your Autumn altar, such as the kitchen or by the fire in your living room.

**1.** Lay out an altar cloth of rich autumnal hues of burnt orange, russet red, rusty yellow. A loose-spun linen is ideal but it could equally be something more homely – perhaps a hand-crocheted or embroidered shawl.

**2.** Light some yellow candles and a dark green one to honour the growth which is descending into the earth.

**3.** Place items which symbolize Autumn: a sheaf of corn, a corn dolly, a wreath of oak leaves, nuts and seeds, pumpkins and gourds.

**4.** Burn earthy, warming scents such as patchouli, pine, cedarwood, or black pepper in an aromatherapy burner.

**5.** Offer up all the things you have decided to clear from your life – items or pictures of people and a letter to yourself, putting down your aims and intentions.

### BAKING BREAD

*There's something miraculous about bread. It's about as earthy as food gets yet is also highly spiritual fare. Baking bread plugs you in with the earth and the energy of harvest and Autumn. It's wonderful if you're feeling irritable or anxious – pounding dough is the best anger therapy! See pages 152-153 for a recipe that makes nutty, earthy, delicious bread.*

# Sunday THANKSGIVING WISHES

Go for a good, brisk walk, whatever the weather! Notice the shifting scenery. Give thanks for all the good things that have happened in the year so far. Even if you live in a town or city, Autumn makes its presence known. If you enjoy your walk, why not decide to make it any every day or every weekend activity?

If you haven't yet mastered the art of good breathing, now is a good time to start (see exercises on pages 19, 26, 40, and 87). In Chinese medicine this time of year is governed partly by the lungs so help your body stave off coughs and infections by breathing fully and well.

This afternoon, consider what you really want or need from life. The Core Statement on page 79 will help you.

## GRATITUDE SUPPER

Prepare a magical meal to celebrate the abundant harvest and the joy of close friends and family. Throughout your supper, focus on the positive and the affirmative.

✦ Choose a menu which makes the most of the colours and tastes of Autumn: a golden chowder of sweetcorn and potato; a rich earthy vegetable and grain stew; a vibrant stirfry or pasta with roasted vegetables. Follow with spiced baked apples; a pecan or pumpkin pie; or delicious pancakes topped with maple syrup.

✦ Take great care with your preparations. Lay the table with a yellow cloth and scatter nuts, seeds, and corn husks on the cloth. Light your table with yellow, red, orange, and dark green candles. Place a large bowl of fruit in the middle of the table.

✦ Make place-cards for each person – perhaps cutting them into the shape of Autumn leaves. Write on the back some of the things you really love and appreciate about the person. Use it as a unique opportunity to thank them.

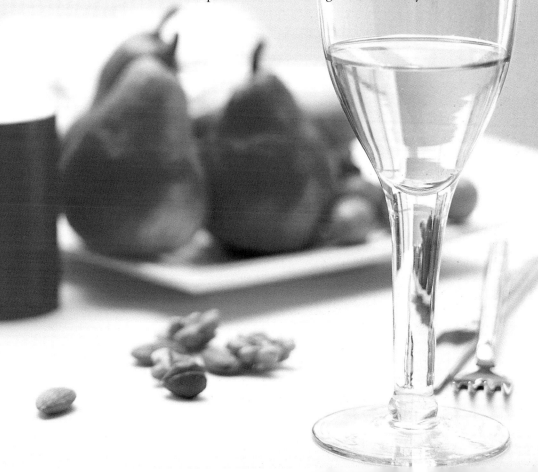

✦ Cook your meal with mindfulness and love. As you cut and chop, stir and season, pour into the food all the wishes and hopes you have for the people who will share your supper. Certain herbs have magical properties: add rosemary for protection and courage; dill for prosperity; and sage for wisdom.

✦ Before you eat, say grace or a blessing – a formal prayer, a time of silent contemplation, or a few spoken words of thanks. You might like to think about the process that has brought this food to your table.

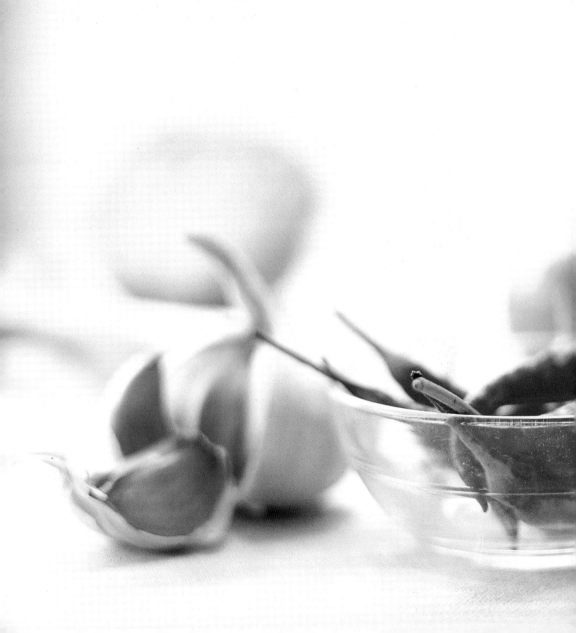

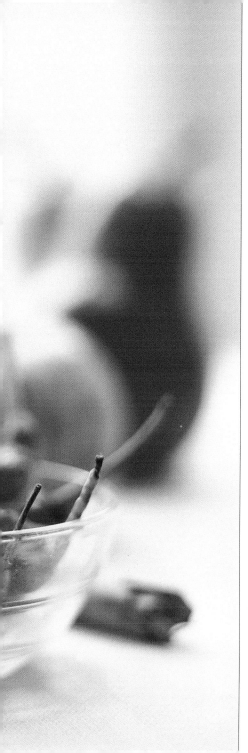

# Welcoming Winter

*Winter may be unwelcoming but there is valid work to be done (and fun to be had, too). It's the time of year when our focus turns inwards and we think about soul work, about seeking spirituality and finding our inner selves. So this is a very important weekend and, if you can, make space for it around the time of the Winter Solstice.*

*WHAT YOU'LL NEED:*
- *Food for Winter (see page 144)*
- *Essential oils: mandarin, pine, and juniper*
- *Sterilized bottles*
- *Other preserve-making equipment and ingredients (optional)*
- *Candles*
- *Tarot cards*
- *Paints, paper (optional)*
- *Your choice of items for your altar*

# Saturday WARMTH AND COMFORT

Give yourself some quiet time to muse about your life and whether you are enjoying it to the full. Ask yourself:

✦ What are my values and beliefs? If I lived them 100 per cent how would that look in my life? How would the people around me react?

✦ What parts of myself do I hide from others for fear of disapproval? What parts do I bury even from myself?

✦ Am I living where and how I want to live, or where and how someone else wants me to live?

✦ What do I need in my life to be free?

Get up, dress warmly, and make a good solid breakfast of porridge/oatmeal or pancakes with maple syrup plus a glass of freshly squeezed orange juice for vitamin C. For lunch, cook a warming soup or stew (curried parsnip and apple, seafood chowder or mulligatawny are soothing).

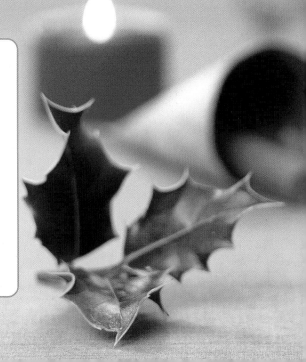

**MAKE A HEARTH**
*If you don't have a hearth, bring in the Fire element with a group of candles in a symbolic hearth – in an unused fireplace or simply in a large metal dish on a table.*

**FOOD FOR WINTER**
*You need a warming and comforting diet to combat chills, fevers, aches, and pains.*
✦ *Eat soups and stews from root vegetables.*
✦ *Eat a little more meat – game is good, totally free range, and low in cholesterol.*
✦ *Keep eating greens (cabbage, kale, leeks, Brussels sprouts).*
✦ *Onions and garlic enhance and strengthen your immune system.*
✦ *Use warming spices and herbs (ginger, cardomom, chilli, cumin, coriander).*
✦ *Stew apples and pears with dried fruits or bake bananas and add honey.*

## WINTER ALTAR

✦ Use a deep green or red cloth (rich and sumptuous like velvet or perhaps a paisley or tartan cloth).

✦ Add to it red and green candles, and leaves of mistletoe and evergreens such as cedar, fir, or holly.

✦ Place a bowl of pot pourri on the altar (with spices such as cinnamon, star anise, pine cones soaked in water with a few drops of cedarwood or sandalwood essential oil). Stud oranges with cloves.

✦ Include photographs of your family – even ones of people who drive you mad – this season is about the people we need rather than those we like!

✦ Add a bell (its ringing cleanses the environment) and Sun symbols to remind you Winter won't last forever.

### ONION SYRUP

*This is marvellous for thick chesty coughs as it helps to loosen phlegm.*
**1.** *Cut 6 large organic onions into chunks and place in a bain-marie. Add ⅓ pint (200 ml) of clear, runny, wild honey. Cover and cook very slowly for around 2 hours.*
**2.** *Strain and bottle in sterilized bottles.*

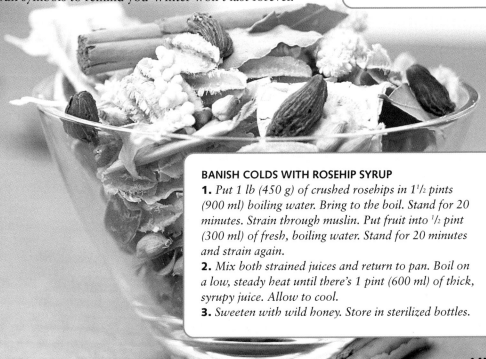

### BANISH COLDS WITH ROSEHIP SYRUP

**1.** *Put 1 lb (450 g) of crushed rosehips in 1½ pints (900 ml) boiling water. Bring to the boil. Stand for 20 minutes. Strain through muslin. Put fruit into ½ pint (300 ml) of fresh, boiling water. Stand for 20 minutes and strain again.*
**2.** *Mix both strained juices and return to pan. Boil on a low, steady heat until there's 1 pint (600 ml) of thick, syrupy juice. Allow to cool.*
**3.** *Sweeten with wild honey. Store in sterilized bottles.*

# Sunday FOCUSING ON THE FUTURE

Once again, get outside for a dose of fresh air and light. Try "prayer walking" like the monks who paced complicated labyrinths to focus their minds on their devotions. If you're feeling really adventurous (and you have a large garden!) you could plan out your own maze or labyrinth (using small stones or gravel paths) but it's not essential! Simply walking is good enough.

Take half an hour for your walk: five minutes to focus your thoughts; at least 15 for the walk itself, and another five to sift through what you've learned. Walk at a comfortable pace but keep up a good rhythm. Think over a scripture, recite a religious mantra, or repeat a word with significance for you – such as "hope" or "peace".

## TAROT REVELATIONS

Winter is the classic time for divination. If you don't already use the Tarot cards, now is a good time to begin. The Tarot cards show universal experiences of life – from birth and innocence, through love and work, to old age and wisdom.

It is important to remember that the Tarot will never tell you what will happen, only what is most likely to happen, given your circumstances and state of mind at the time of the reading. We all have free will and we can all decide how to live our lives: the Tarot simply forewarns us about possible difficulties ahead. Pick a pack which really appeals to you. I usually suggest beginners start with the Rider Waite pack because each card has a pictorial representation which is really helpful – particularly when you're starting out. Take a while to get to know your cards. Look at them, see which cards attract you and which you find unpleasant. People who have problems with relationships might find The Lovers card a difficult image. For others a dislike of authority might make them react with distaste to images such as The Emperor. Simply pondering your reaction to these images may well bring about quite profound insights about your personality.

Picking a Daily Card (see below) is a also brilliant way to begin.

## SOOTHING BATH

Enjoy a soothing bath before going to bed. Add two drops each of pine and juniper oil to a cup of milk and swirl into the bath.

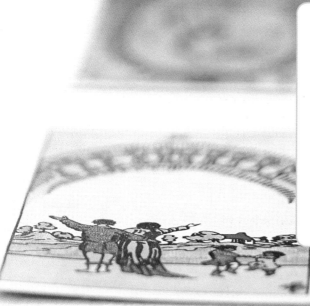

### PICKING A DAILY CARD

✦ *Sit quietly. Breathe slowly and steadily, and focus on your breath. Allow distracting thoughts to slip away.*
✦ *Slowly, mindfully shuffle the Tarot pack. When you feel ready put the pack in front of you. With your left hand, cut three piles towards the left and put them on top of one another.*
✦ *Turn the top card over. This shows the quality of the day ahead. Consider its symbolism, name, colours. Look up its meaning. Think about how it relates to you and your situation.*

# ✿ Sun Salutation

The Sun Salutation is a series of traditional yoga moves which sends a surge of energy and wellbeing throughout your entire body (and mind!). You may find it helpful to record the instructions on a cassette recorder until you are familiar with them.

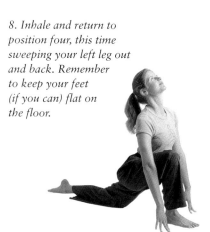

*1. Stand upright and bring your feet together. Relax your shoulders, tuck your chin in slightly, look straight ahead. Bring your hands together in front of your chest with palms together as if you were praying. Exhale deeply.*

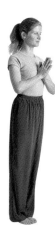

*10. Inhale and return to position one. Exhale as you bring your hands together as a sign of prayer.*

*8. Inhale and return to position four, this time sweeping your left leg out and back. Remember to keep your feet (if you can) flat on the floor.*

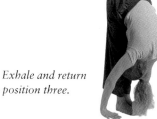

*9. Exhale and return to position three.*

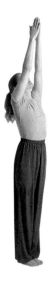

*2. Inhale slowly and deeply while you bring your arms up over your head. Place your palms together as you finish inhaling. Look up at your thumbs. Lift the knees by tightening your thighs. Reach up to lengthen your whole body, but don't overdo it.*

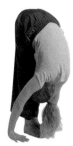

*3. Exhale as you bend forwards so that your hands are beside your feet and your head touching your knees. You may need to bend your knees in order to reach. Eventually you should be able to straighten your knees into the full posture.*

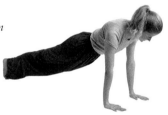

*4. Inhale and sweep your right leg out and back in a kind of extended lunge position. Keep your hands and left foot firmly on the ground. Tilt your head upwards, stretching out your back.*

*5. Exhale and let your left leg join your right and extend your arms to support you. Your hands point forwards, your arms are shoulder-width apart, and your back is in a line with your head and legs. Inhale.*

*7. Inhale and bend up into the cobra position. Bend backwards as far as feels comfortable. Look upwards and exhale.*

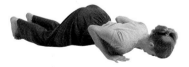

*6. Exhale and lower your body on to the floor. Try to keep your abdomen raised and your nose off the floor so only your forehead makes contact. Don't worry if it seems impossible – just keep the idea in mind.*

**149**

# Moon Salutation

The Moon Salutation is a lovely, relaxing yoga sequence – just right for the end of the day. It takes about five minutes and leaves you balanced and ready for the evening ahead, no matter what you have in store.

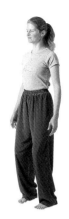

*1. Stand upright, feet shoulder-width apart, knees softly bent, and your arms hanging loosely by your sides. Your head is balanced easily on your neck – you might imagine a string attached to the very top of your head gently pulling you up into alignment.*

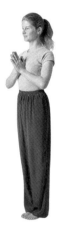

*10. Go back through the sequence to position one, and finish with your hands together as a sign of salutation, known as namaskarasana.*

*9. Inhale gently and bring your torso along the floor by bending your arms and then straightening them, pushing your head, shoulders, and torso back into the Cobra position.*

*8. Exhale gently and bring your arms and torso down and forwards, lowering your buttocks to rest on your calves. Touch your head on the floor and bend forwards into the Tortoise position.*

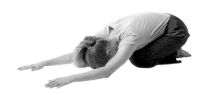

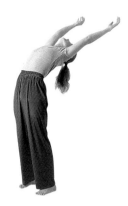

*3. Exhale gently, slowly bringing the arms forwards. Bend your torso forwards, keeping your legs straight, touch the floor with your palms.*

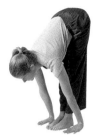

*2. Inhale softly and raise both arms up over the head. Gently bend your upper body and head backwards as far as is comfortable.*

*4. Inhale gently, bend the knees and lower your buttocks slowly into a squat. Exhale.*

*7. Inhale gently and bring your right knee back to rest on the floor beside your left knee. Standing on your knees, raise your arms up over your head and gently bend your body back as far as is comfortable. This is known as the Half Moon position.*

*5. Inhale gently. Extend the left leg back with the knee touching the floor. Raise your arms over your head and bend your upper body back into the pose known as the Flag.*

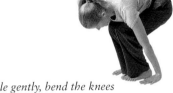

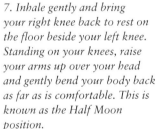

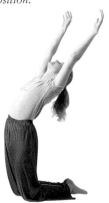

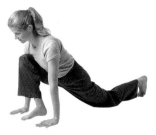

*6. Exhale gently, bringing your palms down to the floor, and stretch your body forward as far as possible into the leg spread.*

**151**

# Recipes

## MOROCCAN CHICKEN
*(serves four)*

4 chicken breasts
2 onions, finely chopped
1 teaspoon of fresh ginger, chopped (or 1 teaspoon of ground)
Salt and black pepper to taste
1 lb (500 g) of sharp eating apples (e.g. Granny Smith), peeled, cored, and sliced. Use pears, prunes, fresh dates, and raisins for variety
2 tablespoons of fresh parsley, finely chopped
1 teaspoon of butter (optional)

Put the chicken, onions, and parsley in a saucepan and cover with water. Add the butter (if used), ginger, and season.

Bring to the boil, cover the pan, and allow to simmer until the chicken is tender and the onions are almost disintegrated, making a reduced sauce. This should take about 40 mins to an hour. Add the apples and allow to simmer again until they are tender but not disintegrated.

Serve with your choice of brown rice, couscous, or bread.

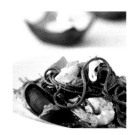

## ROMANTIC SPAGHETTI
*(serves two)*

5.5 oz (150 g) black spaghetti
1 tablespoon of olive oil
2 cloves of garlic, chopped not crushed
13 oz (350 g) of plum tomatoes, skinned and chopped
$\frac{1}{2}$ teaspoon of sugar
5.5 oz (150 g) of shelled prawns
12 mussels in their shells
5.5 oz (150 g) fillet of salmon, sliced
One medium-sized squid, sliced into rounds
Basil leaves, chopped

Stir fry the garlic in oil for a few seconds and add tomatoes. Stir for 5-10 mins into a sauce. Cook mussels for 4 mins (discard shells that don't open when cooked) first and the rest of the seafood for 2-4 mins. Mix seafood, sauce, sugar, and salt/pepper to taste.

Add the spaghetti to a pan of boiling salted water, following instructions on packet. Mix the spaghetti and sauce, sprinkle the fresh basil on top, and serve.

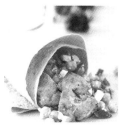

## SUMMER PICNIC
*(serves six)*

### Chicken Marinade:
$\frac{2}{3}$ pint (400 ml) yoghurt
1 tablespoon coriander, chopped
A pinch of chilli powder
1 teaspoon cumin powder
1 teaspoon garam masala

Thoroughly mix the marinade with six chicken breasts, cover and leave for 2-3 hours in the fridge. Grill the chicken or barbecue it on a skewer until nicely golden.

### Chickpea and Feta Salad:
17.5 oz (480 g) cooked chickpeas
6.5 oz (180 g) of feta cheese (Greek not Danish)
A handful of chopped flat-leaved parsley
14.5 oz (400 g) of fresh tomatoes, sliced
Dressing (3 parts olive oil to 1 part lemon juice)
Seasoning

Mix the salad and serve in wraps or pitta bread with the chicken on top.

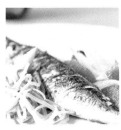

## ENERGY FISH DISH
*(serves two)*

2 medium-sized mackerel
1 fennel, finely sliced
1 pink grapefruit
1 cucumber, finely sliced and lightly seasoned
A handful of black olives
Seasoning
Salt

Buy mackerel cleaned and beheaded from a reputable fishmonger. Use supermarkets as a last resort. For the best taste, find mackerel that have been landed that day or at least in the last 24-36 hours – the rainbow colours on the skin should dazzle. If the colour is dull, then don't bother.

Sprinkle a little salt on the skin before grilling at a high heat; 5-8 mins each side should suffice.

Serve with a cucumber salad plus a salad of finely sliced raw fennel and segmented pink grapefruit that has been tossed with a few black olives, the juice from the grapefruit, and seasoning.

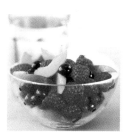

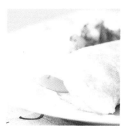

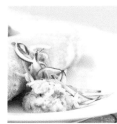

### DETOX FRUIT SALAD
*(serves two)*

*18 oz (500 g) apricots, fresh*
*9 oz (250 g) raspberries*
*9 oz (250 g) blueberries*
*A few green cardamon seeds*
*²/₃ pint (400 ml) of yoghurt*

*Slice apricots and mix with raspberries and blueberries. Stir the cardamon seeds (remove the seeds by breaking open the pods) into the yoghurt and serve.*

*Other suggestions: Swap apricots for fresh figs and also use peaches, blackberries, blackcurrants, damsons, mulberries, and mangos.*

### DOSA PANCAKES
*(serves four)*

*1 cup of cornmeal*
*1 cup of rice flour*
*2-3 cups of just boiled water*
*A large pinch of sea salt*
*¹/₂ teaspoon of olive oil or ghee*

*Mix the cornmeal, flour, water, and salt thoroughly but you don't need to beat or whisk. Cover and leave overnight.*
*Put about half a teaspoon of oil or ghee in a non-stick frying pan and heat until hot. Pour in a small amount of mixture and gently spread with the back of a spoon in a spiral motion until you have a dosa about 4-6 ins (10-15 cms) in diameter. Allow to brown then flip over onto the other side. Keep it warm while you make the rest of the dosas.*

**Coriander chutney:**
*Serve with a chutney made from freshly chopped coriander, grated coconut, and a small amount of chopped mint in yoghurt.*

### MASALA POTATOES
*(serves four)*

*4 potatoes, cubed and parboiled*
*2 tablespoons of oil*
*2 fl. oz (50 ml) of water*
*¹/₄ teaspoon of turmeric*
*1 teaspoon of curry powder*
*1 teaspoon of onion seeds*
*1 tomato, chopped*
*Garlic, chilli, green cumin, and coriander*
*Lemon juice (optional)*
*1 teaspoon of sea salt*

*Heat the oil and add the onion seeds, tomato, and finely chopped garlic, ginger, a pinch of chilli, green cumin, and freshly chopped coriander.*
*Reduce heat and cook for 3 minutes. Stir in the potatoes, lemon juice, salt, and water. Cook together for 15 mins. until the potatoes are tender*
*You can serve as a separate dish or wrapped in a dosa pancake to make a Masala dosa.*

### BAKING BREAD

*2.2 lbs (1 kg) of granary malted flour*
*A small handful of yeast*
*1 pint (²/₃ litre) of warm water*
*1 teaspoon of sugar*
*¹/₂ tablespoon of sea salt*
*2 tablespoons of olive oil*

*Put a small handful of yeast into a bowl and add a teaspoon of sugar and a little of the warm water (from a measured pint). Mix until you hear it bubble. Set your oven to gas mark 6 or 180° C.*
*Put the granary malted flour into another bowl. Scatter the sea salt over the flour and add the olive oil. Now add the rest of the warm water.*
*Pour the yeast mix over the flour mixture. Squeeze and knead the dough together.*
*Leave the bread to rise in a warm spot for 10 mins. Break into rolls (if you're feeling clever you could plait them or make mini cottage loaves). Bake for 20-24 mins. To test, take one out and tap the bottom: if it sounds hollow then it's done.*
*Now all you have to do is eat the rolls (with a hearty bowl of soup) for your supper.*

**153**

# Resources

Please send an SAE when writing to these organizations. Many have on-line registers of practitioners, so do check their websites first to save time and administration.

The National Institute of Ayurvedic Medicine
584 Milltown Road
Brewster, NY 10509
drgerson@erols.com
www.niam.com
Tel: (914) 278-8700
Fax: (914) 278-8700

American Association of Naturopathic
Physicians
601 Valley Street, Suite 105
Seattle, WA 98109
www.naturopathic.org
Tel: (206) 298-0126
Fax: (206) 298-0129

American Naturopathic Medical Association
P.O. Box 96273
Las Vegas, NV 89193
www.webmaster@anma.com
Tel: (702) 897-7053

American Association of Nutrition Consultants
1641 East Sunset Road
Apt. B-117
Las Vegas, NV 89119
Tel: (709) 361-1132

American Yoga Association
P.O. Box 19986
Sarasota, FL 34276
info@americanyogaassociation.org
www.americanyogaassociation.org
Tel: (941) 927-4977
Fax: (941) 921-9844

American Oriental Bodywork Therapy
Association
50 Maple Street
Manhasset, NY 11030

International School of Shiatsu
10 South Clinton Street
Doylestown, PA 18901
info@shiatsubo.com
www.shiatsubo.com
Tel: (215) 340-9918
Fax: (215) 340-9181

American Massage Therapy Association
820 Davis Street
Suite 100
Evanston, IL 96201-4444
www.amtamassage.org
Tel: (847) 864-0123
Fax: (847) 864-1178

American Alliance of Aromatherapy
P.O. Box 309
Depoe Bay, OR 97341

International Institute of Reflexology
P.O. Box 12642
St. Petersburg, FL 33733-2642
www.mitcm.org
Tel: (301) 718-7373 and (800) 892-1209
Fax: (301) 718-0735

American Herbalists Guild
P.O. Box 70
Roosevelt, UT 84066
Tel: (435) 722-8434
Fax: (435) 722-8452

American Institute of Homeopathy
1585 Glencoe Street
Suite 44
Denver, CO 80220
Tel: (303) 321-4105

American Feng Shui Institute
108 North Ynez Avenue
Suite 202
Monterey Park, CA 91754
www.amfengshui.com
fsinfor@amfengshui.com
Tel: 626-571-2757
Fax: 626-571-2065

Feng Shui Emporium
1833 Seminole Trail
Charlottesville, VA 22901
www.fengshuiemporium.com
Tel: (434) 973-7223 and (800) 443-5894
Fax: (434) 973-7294

American Meditation Institute
P.O. Box 430
Averill Park, NY 12018
www.americanmeditation.org
Tel: (518) 674-8714

American Counseling Association
5999 Stevenson Avenue
Alexandria, VA 22304-9800
Tel: (703) 823-0988

Association for Humanistic Psychology
45 Franklin Street
Suite 315
San Francisco, CA 94102
www.ahpweb.org
Tel: (415) 864-0885

Sound Healers Association
P.O. Box 2240
Boulder, CO 80306
www.healingsounds.com
Tel: (303) 443-8181
Fax: (303) 443-6023

American Music Therapy Association, Inc.
8455 Colesville Road
Suite 1000
Silver Spring, MD 20910
www.musictherapy.org
Tel: (301) 589-3300

American Art Therapy Association
1202 Allanson Road
Mundelein, IL 60060-3808
www.arttherapy.org
Tel: (888) 290-0878 and (847) 949-6064
Fax: (847) 566-4580

Jane Alexander's website at www.smudging.com provides information on a wide range of mind, body, spirit topics.

# Further reading

These books are useful background reading for each weekend.

## BODY AWARENESS
Alexander, J, **The Five Minute Healer**, Gaia, 2000
Shapiro, D, **Your Body Speaks your Mind**, Piatkus, 1996
Weller, S, **The Breath Book**, Thorsons, 1999
Golten, R, **The Owner's Guide to the Body**, Thorsons, 1999
Ferguson, P, **The Self-Shiatsu Handbook**, Newleaf, 1996

## DETOX
Alexander, J, **The Detox Plan**, Gaia, 1998
Sabatini, S, **Breath**, Thorsons, 2000
Wheater, C, **Juicing for Health**, Thorsons, 1993
Marshall-Warren, D, **Mind Detox**, Thorsons, 1999
MacDonald Baker, Dr S, **Detoxification & Healing**, Keats, 1997

## ENERGIZING
Alexander, J, **The Energy Secret**, Thorsons, 2000
Hartvig, K and Rowley, Dr N, **You are What you Eat**, Piatkus, 1996
Olivier, S, **Maximising Energy**, Pocket Books, 2000
Proto, L, **Increase your Energy**, Piatkus, 1998
Wills, J, **4 Weeks to Total Energy**, Quadrille, 2000

## BEAUTY
Muryn, M, **Water Magic**, Bantam, 1997
Vyas, B, **Beauty Wisdom**, Thorsons, 1997
Raichur, P, **Absolute Beauty**, Bantam, 1998
Leigh, M, **The New Beauty**, Newleaf, 1996
Antczak, Dr S and G, **Cosmetics Unmasked**, Thorsons, 2001

## AYURVEDA
Alexander, J, **Live Well**, Thorsons, 2001
Morrison, J, **The Book of Ayurveda**, Gaia, 1995
Morningstar, A and Desai, U, **The Ayurvedic Cookbook**, Lotus Light, 1990
Lad, V, **The Complete Book of Ayurvedic Home Remedies**, Piatkus, 1999
Douillard, J, **Body, Mind and Sport**, Harmony, 1994
Pegrum, Juliet, **Vastu Vidya: the Indian art of placement**, Gaia Books, 2000.

## BREAK THE ROUTINE
Levine, S, **A Year to Live**, Thorsons, 1997
Kundtz, D, **Stopping**, Newleaf, 1999
Franks, L, **The Seed Handbook**, Thorsons, 2000
Williams, N, **The Work we were Born to Do**, Element, 1999
James, J, **Reinvent Your Life**, Hodder & Stoughton, 1996

## REARRANGING
Kingston, K, **Clear your Clutter with Feng Shui**, Piatkus, 1998
Rossbach, S, **Interior Design with Feng Shui**, Rider, 1987
Spear, W, **Feng Shui made Easy**, Thorsons, 1995
Linn, D, **Space Clearing**, Ebury Press, 2000
Harrold, F, **Be Your Own Life Coach**, Hodder & Stoughton, 2000

## RELATIONSHIPS
Davies, Dr B, **Affairs of the Heart**, Hodder & Stoughton, 2000
Richardson, D, **The Love Keys**, Element, 1999
Eason, C, **A Magical Guide to Love & Sex**, Piatkus, 2000
Resnick, S, **The Pleasure Zone**, Newleaf, 1997

## EXPLORE YOUR SUBCONSCIOUS

Schneider, M and Killick, J, **Writing for Self-Discovery**, Element, 1998

Weiss, L, **Practical Dreaming**, New Harbinger Publications, 1999

Frings Keys, M, **Inward Journey**, Open Court, 1983

Johnson, R, **Owning your Own Shadow**, Thorsons, 1991

Zweig, C & Wolf, S, **Romancing the Shadow**, Thorsons, 1997

## SPIRITUAL AWARENESS

Alexander, J, **Mind Body Spirit**, Carlton, 2001

Weston, W, **How Prayer Heals**, Hampton Roads, 1998

Ostrom, J, **Auras**, Thorsons, 2000

Judith, A, **Eastern Body, Western Mind**, Celestial Arts, 1996

## RETREAT

Louden, J, **The Woman's Retreat Book**, HarperSanFrancisco, 1997

Goldman, J, **Healing Sounds**, Element, 1992

Alexander, J, **Spirit of the Home**, Thorsons, 1998

Owens, E, **Women Celebrating Life**, Llewellyn, 2000

Robertson, R & J, **The Sacred Kitchen**, New World Library, 1999

## QABALAH

Crowley, V, **A Woman's Kabbalah**, Thorsons, 2001

Parfitt, W, **The Living Qabalah**, Element, 1988

Ashcroft-Nowicki, D, **Inner Landscapes**, Aquarian, 1989

Ashcroft-Nowicki, D, **First Steps in Ritual**, Aquarian, 1982

Jayanti, A, **The Qabalah**, Thorsons, 1999

## SHAMANISM

Alexander, J, **The Smudge Pack**, Thorsons, 1999

Rutherford, L, **Shamanism**, Thorsons, 1996

Matthews, C, **Singing the Soul Back Home**, Element, 1995

Bates, B, **The Wisdom of the Wyrd**, Rider, 1996

## SEASONS

Linn, D, **Altars**, Ebury Press, 1999

Streep, P, **Altars Made Easy**, HarperCollins, 1997

Alexander, J, **Sacred Rituals at Home**, Sterling, 2000

Bartimeus, P, **Eating with the Seasons**, Element, 1998

Hamaker-Zondag, K, **The Way of the Tarot**, Piatkus, 1998

# Index

BOSTON PUBLIC LIBRARY

3 9999 04437 819 6

GL

BAKER & TAYLOR